The Spirit of Botany

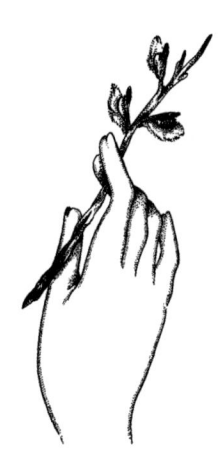

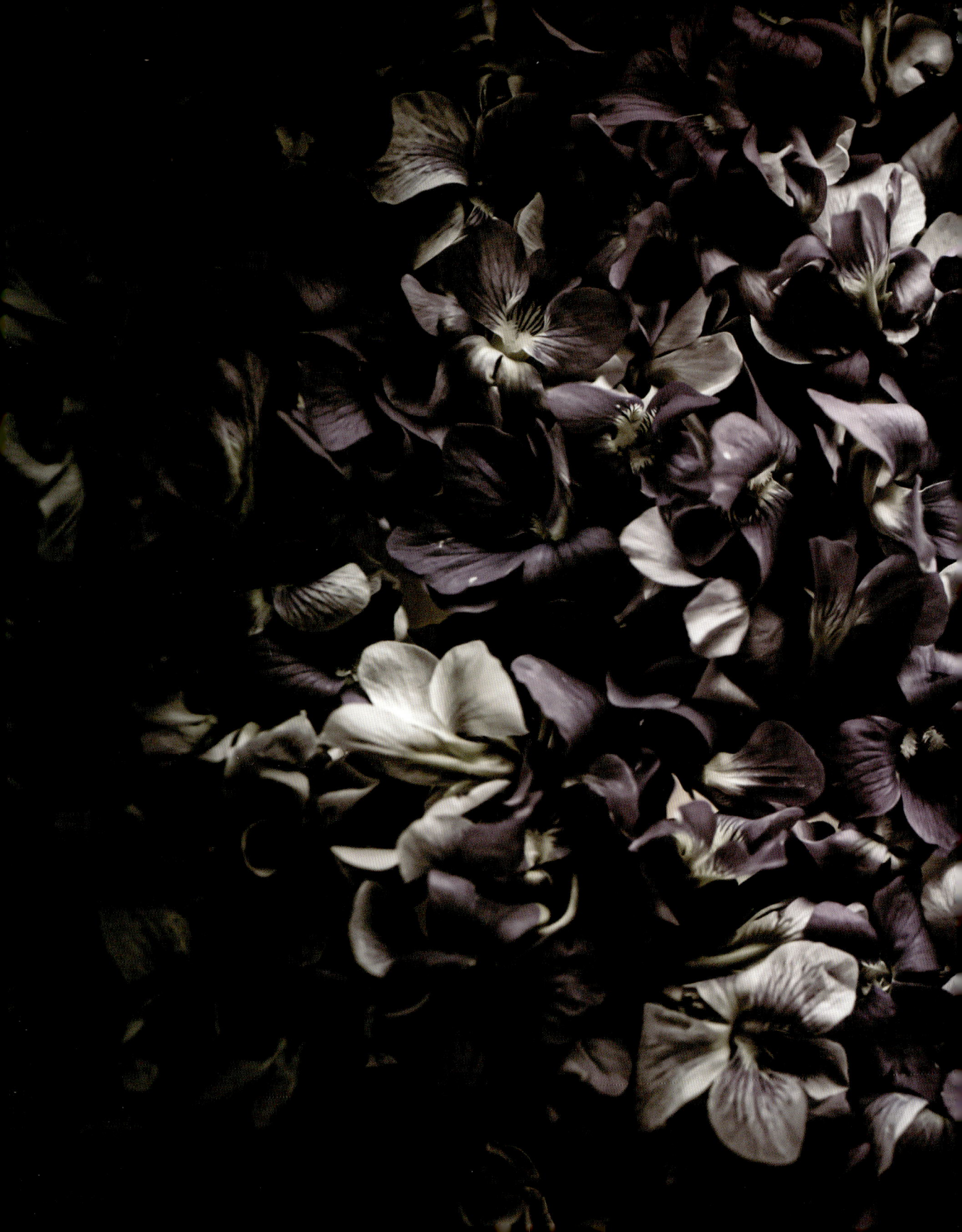

THE SPIRIT OF BOTANY

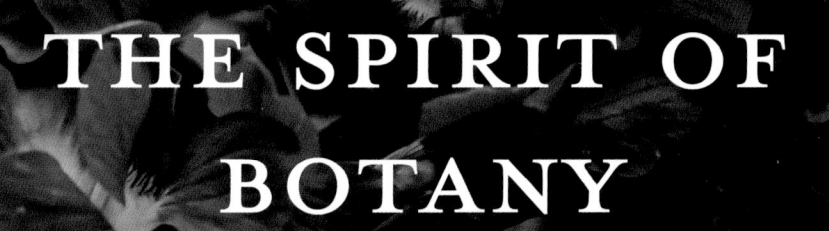

Aromatic Recipes and Rituals

JILL M^cKEEVER

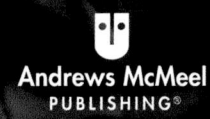

Andrews McMeel
PUBLISHING®

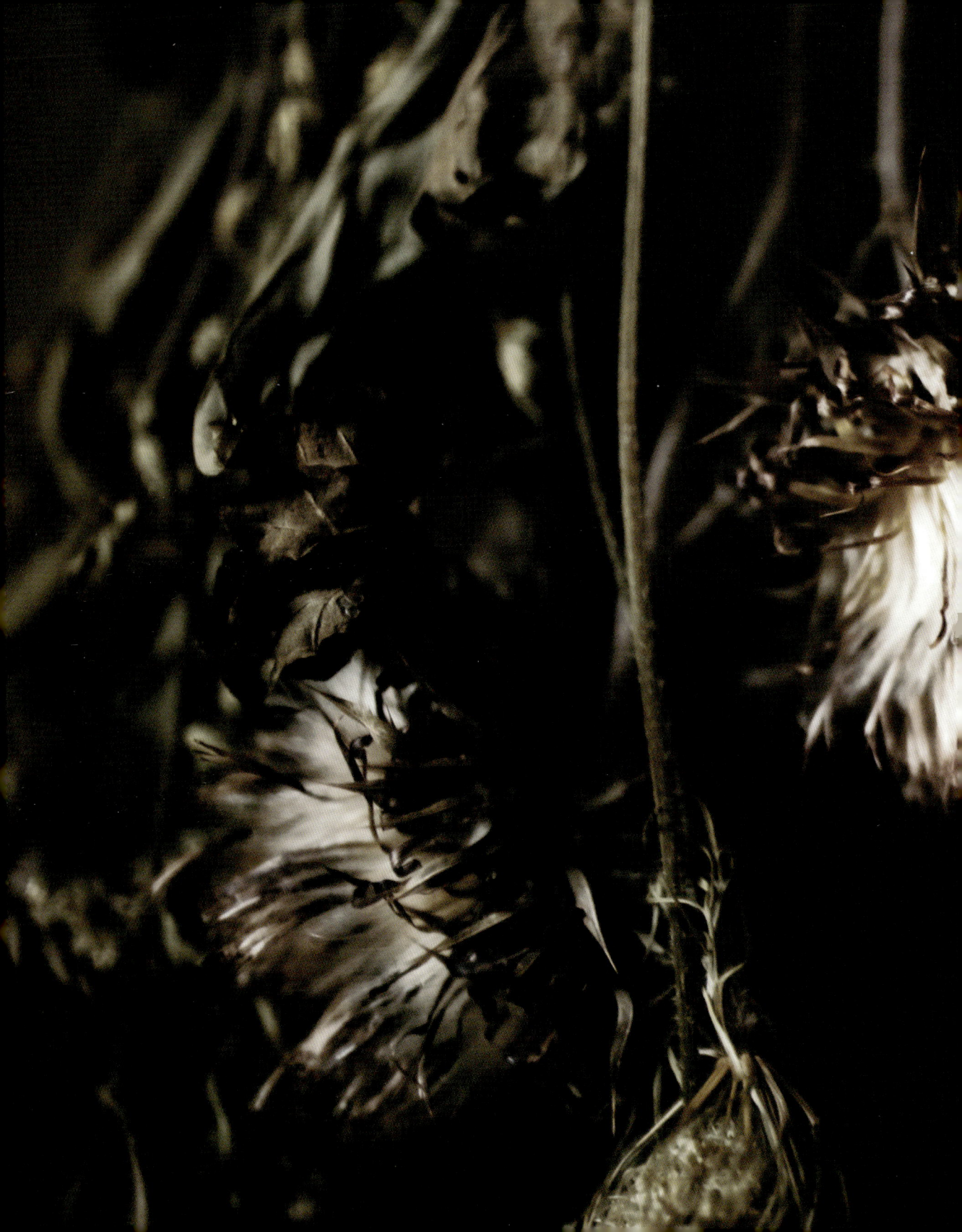

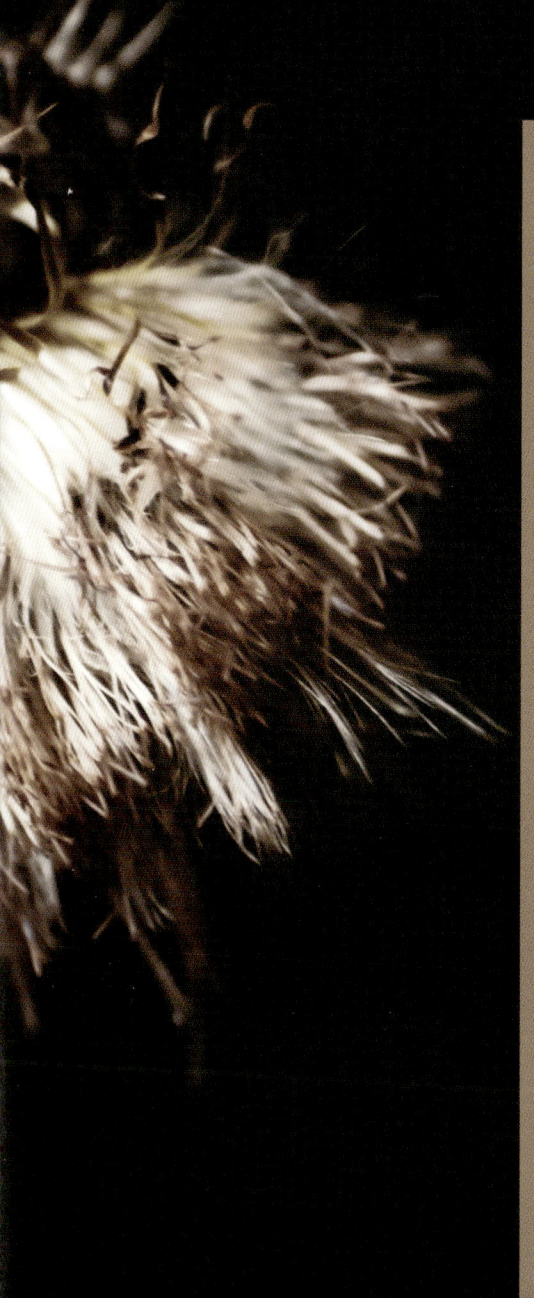

Contents

ABOUT THIS BOOK   IX

One | MY STORY   1

Two | ESSENTIAL OILS   11

Three | BOTANICAL PERFUME   21

Four | SYNESTHESIA   27

Five | BOTANICAL MATERIALS   33

Six | INCENSE   69

Seven | WELCOMING THE SEASONS   79

Eight | THE MOON   93

Nine | AROMATHERAPY   101

Ten | DREAM WORK   119

Eleven | NATURE THERAPY   131

GOODBYE   135

ACKNOWLEDGMENTS   139

ABOUT THE AUTHOR   140

INDEX   142

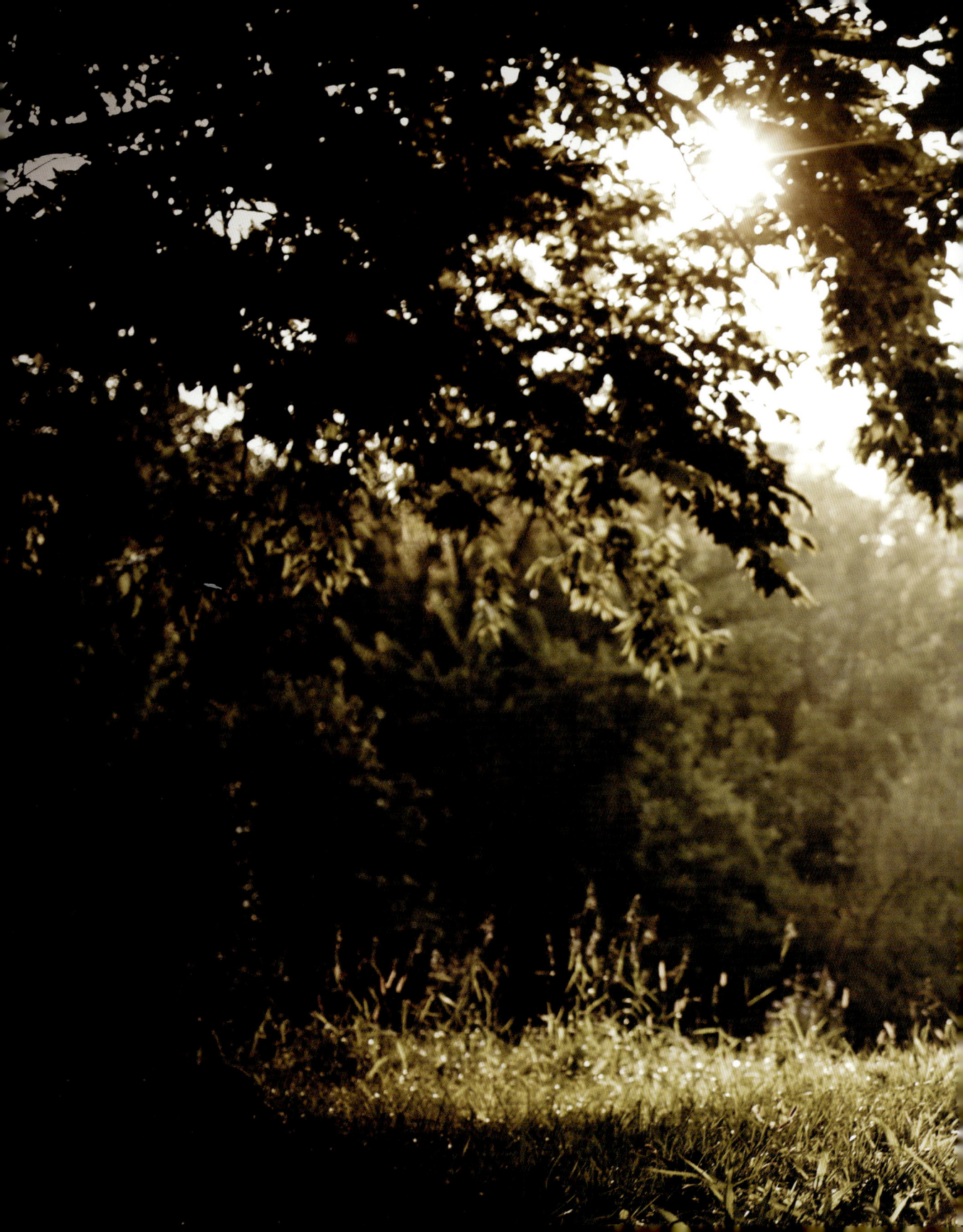

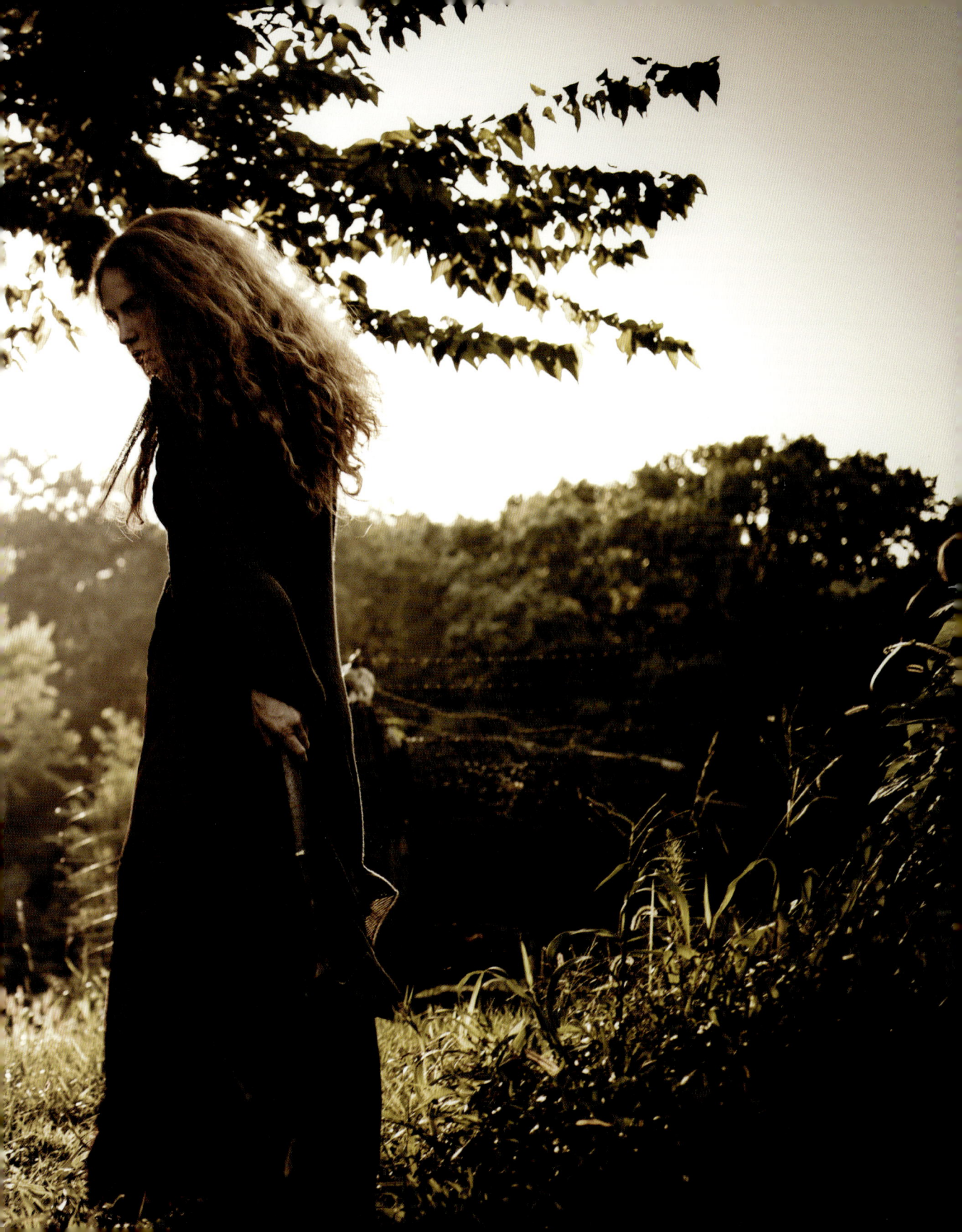

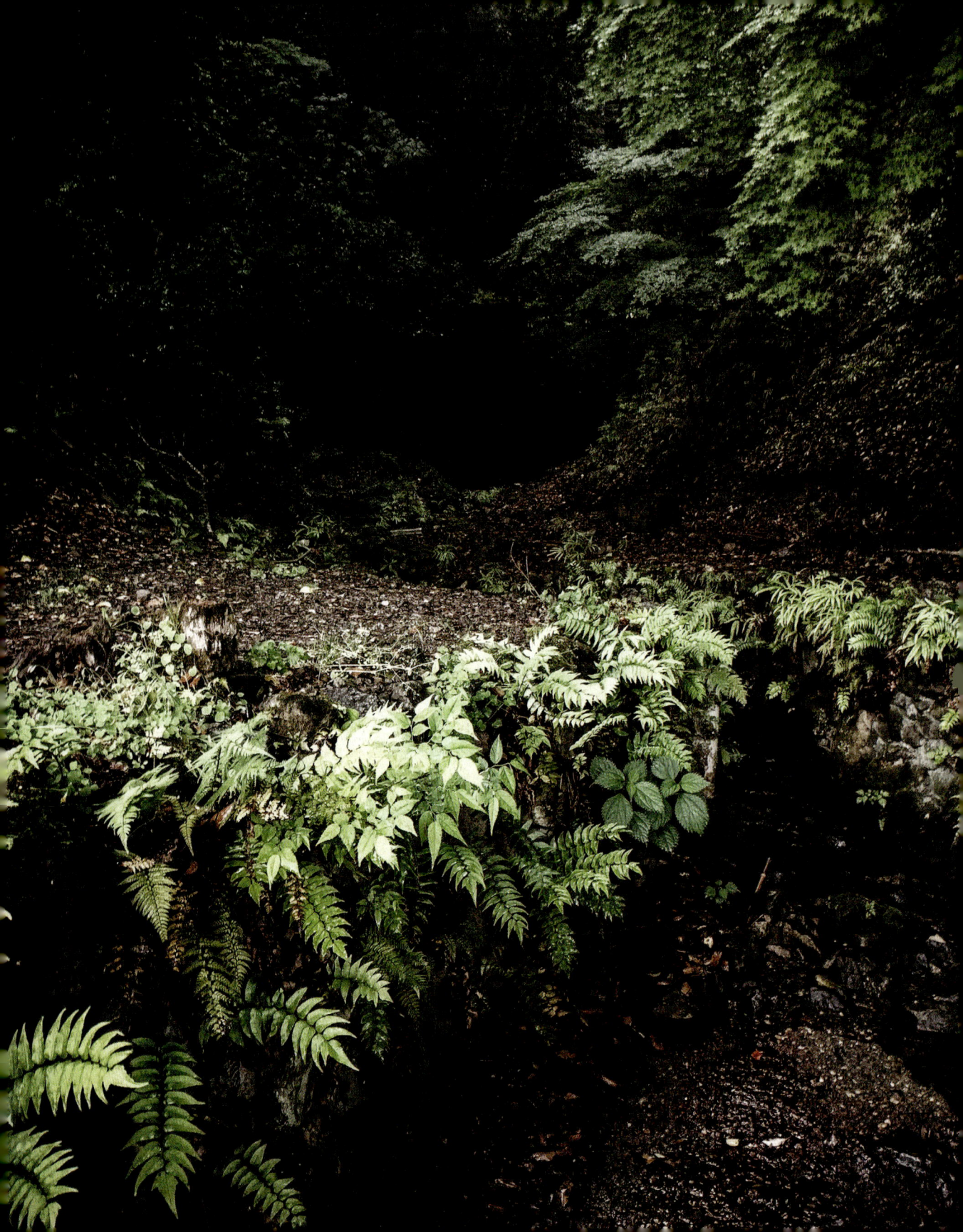

About This Book

The Spirit of Botany is intended for anyone seeking a deeper connection to nature through their senses. It's an exploration of botanical aromatics and their effects on the mind as I have experienced them in my life and work. The energies of plants can hold significant meanings and induce deeply visceral responses. This book is a collection of methods and recipes I've developed through alchemical experiments in my home and studio, using materials that are nothing less than magical.

Developing a personal relationship with the natural environment is essential to understanding ourselves. Many of us live our entire lives in cities covered in concrete, which suppress the nourishment of the earth in favor of the conveniences and values of modern society. It can be very difficult to leave this construct, but there are ways to bring the elements of nature back into our lives, even if we live in an urban environment.

The stories and recipes in this book are focused mainly on aromatherapy—a topic I have been exploring for over a decade in my work as a natural perfumer. Some of the methods used in these recipes may require some extra research if you are a beginner, and some of the materials may be difficult to source. I intend to keep many of these materials available at forstrangewomen.com and provide links to other recommended sources.

Above all, my hope is that something in these pages helps you to understand your senses and mind in a new way, broadening your sensory awareness in the realm of aromatics.

꒰꒱

The information in The Spirit of Botany *is not intended to treat, diagnose, cure, or prevent any disease. It is provided for your information only and may not be construed as medical advice or instruction. No action or inaction should be taken based solely on the contents of this information; instead, readers should consult appropriate health professionals on any matter relating to their health and well-being.*

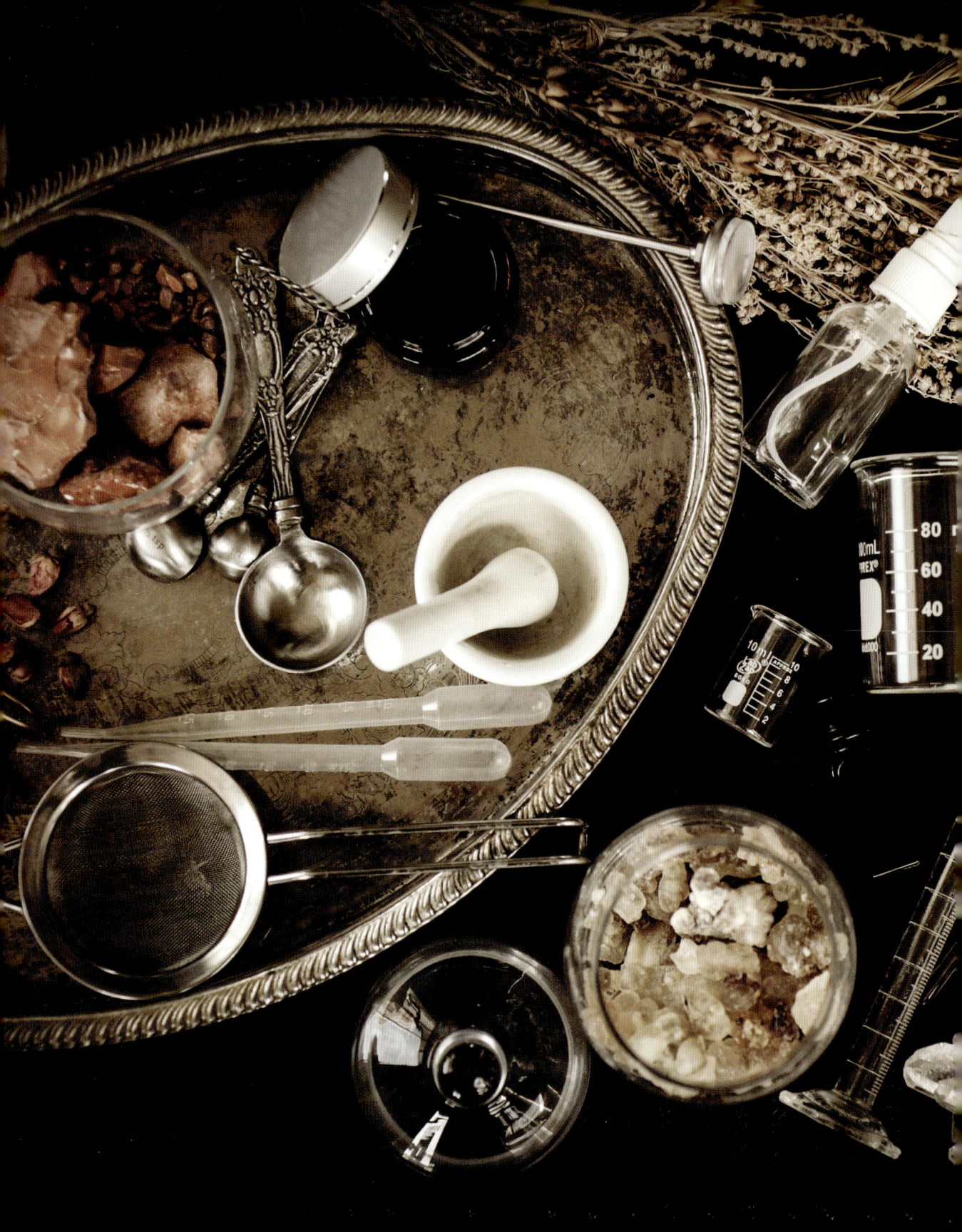

TOOLS YOU'LL NEED

Before creating one of the recipes in this book, you'll want to make sure you have the right tools on hand. As a general rule, choose amber or cobalt glass bottles for storage.

Mortar and pestle (or suribachi)

Kitchen scale

Measuring spoons and cups

Small pipettes for measuring milliliters

Heat-safe glass liquid measuring cup or beaker (small)

Double boiler

Cooking thermometer

Fine-mesh strainer or cheesecloth

Coffee filters

Tea strainer or gaiwan tea set

French press

Funnel (3 to 5 inches wide)

1 and 2-ounce jars or tins with lids

Lip balm tubes (.15 ounce) or tins (.25 ounce)

5-milliliter glass bottle with airtight lid

8, 12, and 16-ounce mason jars

1 and 8-ounce glass bottles with fine-mist sprayers

16-ounce spray bottle (plastic or glass)

Labels

Bakhoor incense burner (and charcoal)

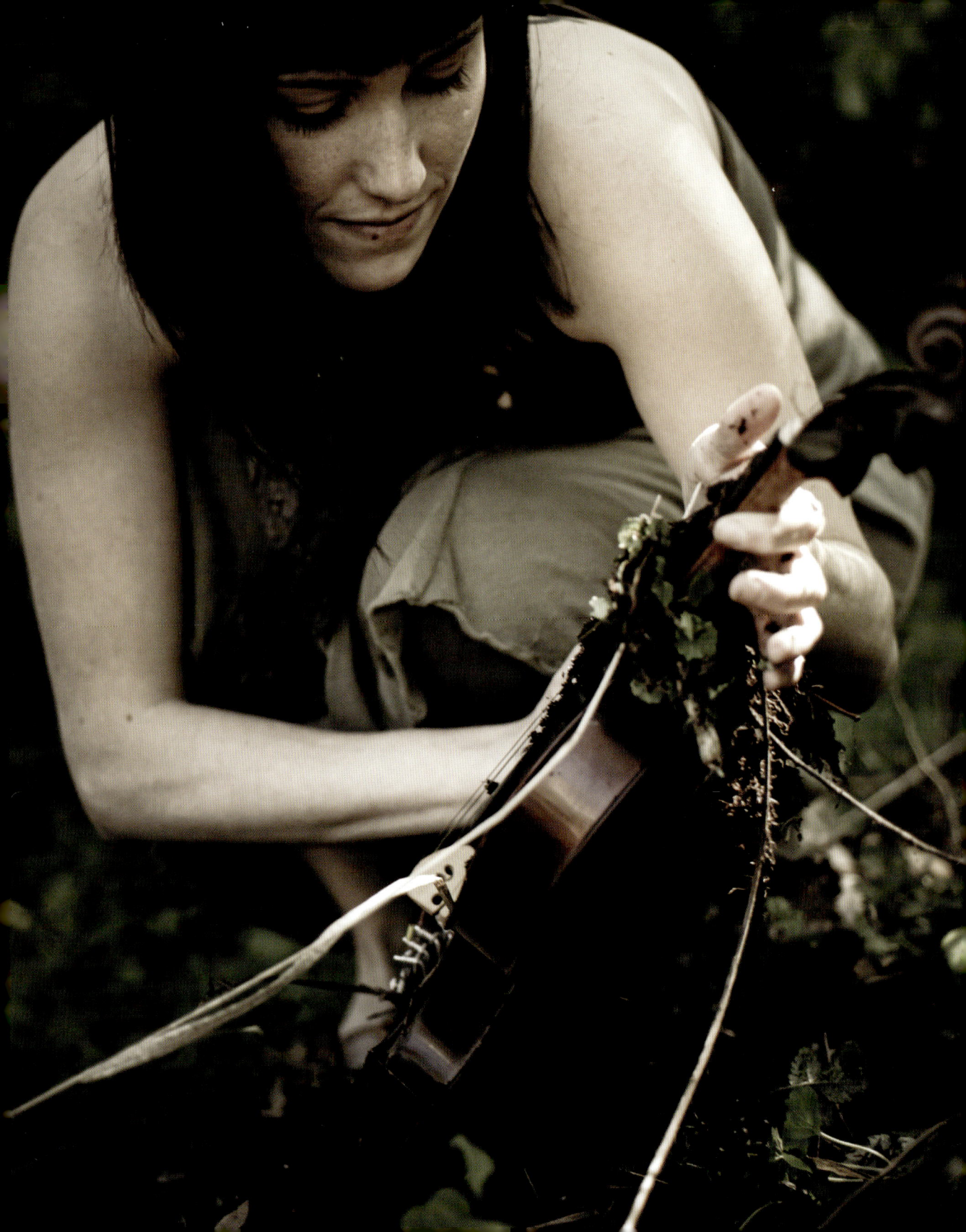

One

MY STORY

I have loved exploring nature since as far back as I can remember. As a child, I was fascinated by insects, seeds, herbs, trees, and animals. I was intrinsically drawn to dance and music, as the energies of these arts also felt like a part of nature to me. When I wasn't running around in the outdoors, discovering all that was alive, I was tracing invisible pathways through space with my body, bringing a new dimension of the music I loved to life through my dancing.

Since then, my creative energy has guided me in many other directions, including photography, film production, music production, and graphic design. My work has been shaped by supportive guides and serendipitous connections, several years of living below the poverty line, and, often, a punk attitude. It has been developed by the beauty and talent of those who surround me, my uncontrolled curiosity, psychedelic plants, and a strong dependence on intuition. It has also been derailed by alcohol, trauma, and even success itself. For a time, I even lost my connection to dance and music, as the pressures of finding my place in the world (a common dilemma for artists) depressed my inspiration. But when I discovered botanical perfume, the interaction with sublimely extracted aromatics brought me back into my body, which is why working as a perfume artist has been my focus now for over a decade.

When I was a teenager, my Catholic mother enrolled me in two years of classes to be confirmed into the church. Looking back, I realize I took the confirmation process a lot more seriously than the other kids my age, believing that once I became formally indoctrinated, I would no longer be free to choose my religion. And so, during those two years, I researched every religion and esoteric spiritual philosophy I could before it was "too late." Although it was fascinating to learn about the perspectives of so many cultures in my search, I did not come to any definite conclusion. Nothing seemed to fit. On the day before my confirmation ceremony, I informed the church that I did not want to be Catholic. That night, I isolated myself in my room (which doubled as a shrine to the Smashing Pumpkins), opened a journal, and wrote that I wanted to "find my own version of god."

At that time, I worked at a craft supplies store, and that week I decided to get the materials to make soap at home. The only problem was that the synthetic soap scents at the store were terrible and gave me headaches. Then, a customer buying soap supplies told me there was this place on the internet where you could purchase *real* essential oils. In the year 2000, this was a whole new concept! I ordered the oils, and upon opening the bottles, I began to feel that connection to the spirit realm I had been hoping to find.

Throughout history and in every culture, humans have intuitively utilized aromatic plants to bridge their connection to the divine. Incense has been used to invite spirits and connect to enlightened states, ritual baths for spiritual protection, infused anointing oils to heal and sanctify, and essential oils have even been buried in tombs for the departed to carry

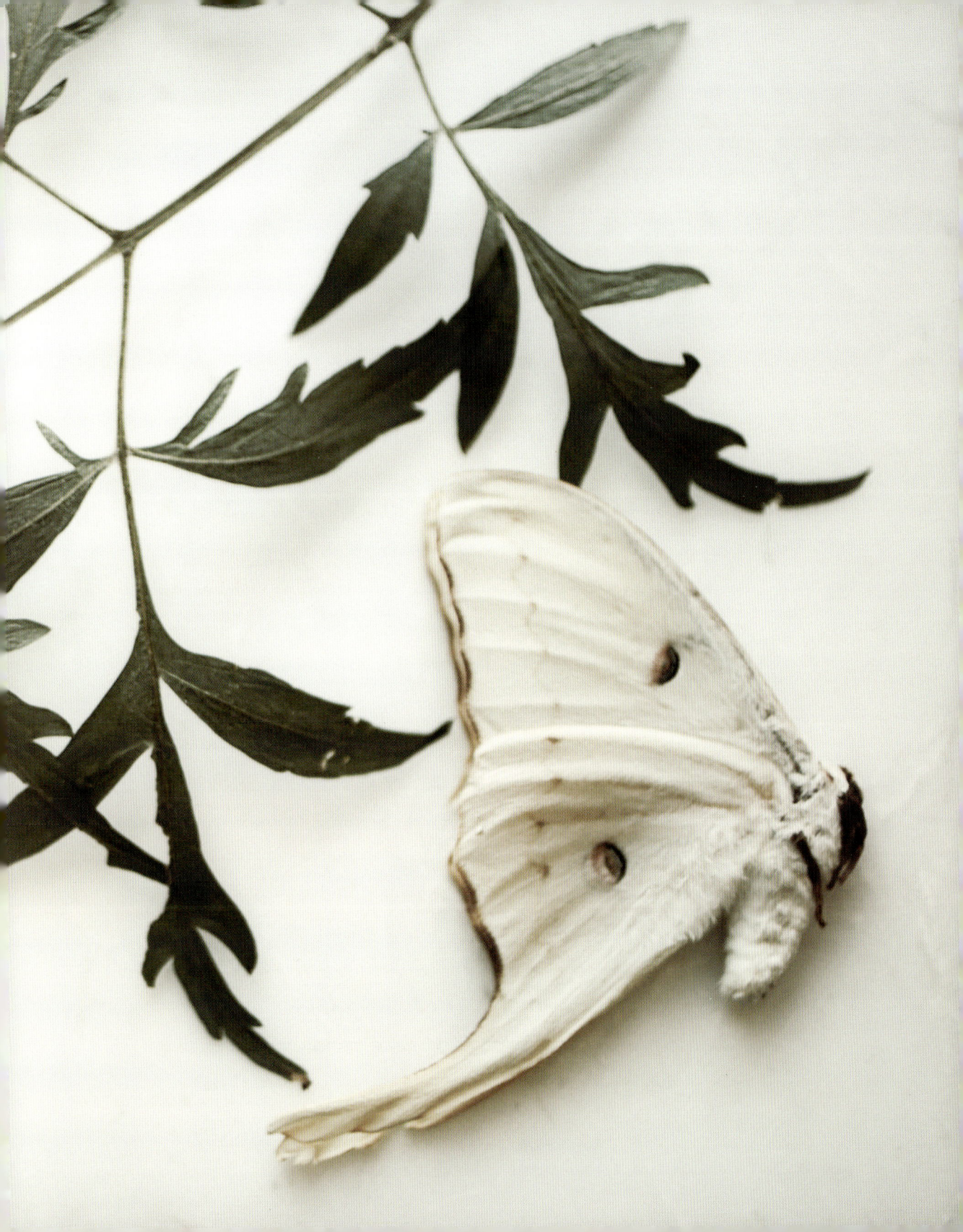

into the afterlife. These methods have all been used in various rituals of protection, purification, healing, and invocation. There may be a lot of different religious and spiritual philosophies in the world, but I have yet to find one that does not use the aromatic spirits of botany to connect to the goddess/universe/enlightenment.

My work as a perfumer began nearly ten years after my introduction to essential oils. It started as a creative outlet I adopted to soothe myself during a couple of years of stressful compromise. I was working as a graphic designer in a communications office in a conservative suburb of Kansas City. The environment was soul crushing, but I desperately needed the paycheck. This was during the Great Recession, and I had purchased a house right before the market collapsed. I found myself far underwater on my mortgage and unable to rely on anyone else for support.

During an internet deep dive, I discovered online communities for the very niche and mysterious realm of botanical perfume. My love for the natural world and the obscure led me to begin sourcing and collecting beautifully extracted aromatics beyond the basic essential oils. I developed an appreciation for the intricacies of these essences and how the molecules recombined as they met with each other. Learning to combine them aesthetically was satisfying in the same way that music and sound production had been for me during my early twenties and that dancing had been when I was a teenager. It was a meditation that brought me back from dissociation, a practice that delivered me into my senses, mind, and body.

Some days at work, I would experience an overwhelming sense of panic. I could feel the electromagnetic energy of the computers buzzing in my head. "I'm not built for this," I would think. During one such episode, I reached into my purse and found a natural perfume blend that I had made at home. The label read "A Tincture for Strange Women." I applied the scent and was instantly transported. I was no longer in the office. I was in Northern California, where the ocean makes the air taste like salt, the wind carries jasmine and rosemary and seaweed to my lungs, and my mind knows it is free from the pressure to conform.

When I began making perfume as an escape, I realized that it was a powerful therapeutic tool as well as a beautiful aesthetic medium, and I wanted to share it. I have been lucky that this work has continued to grow organically over the years and that I am still learning and growing with it.

I still have the original bottle of "A Tincture for Strange Women" in my studio. The scent is composed mainly of top notes, so it doesn't have the depth and complexity that I later developed in my perfume technique. But for the short time this aroma lasts, it is liberating. Top notes give a perfume a sense of expansion and escape, of freedom and energy—exactly what I needed when I created this blend.

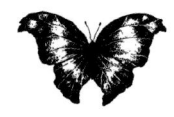

TINCTURE FOR STRANGE WOMEN

Makes 1 ounce of perfume

KOMBU TINCTURE

2 tablespoons dried kombu (kelp)

1 tablespoon assorted botanicals, such as fresh jasmine blooms, lavender buds, and rosemary (optional)

2 ounces 190-proof alcohol

PERFUME

2 milliliters* pink grapefruit essential oil

1 milliliter rosemary essential oil

1 milliliter frankincense essential oil

1 milliliter lavender essential oil

1 milliliter bergamot essential oil

1 milliliter jasmine absolute (Jasminum grandiflorum)*
or ylang-ylang essential oil

* To measure in milliliters, I recommend using a small pipette. You can also measure ¼ teaspoon or about 30 drops as 1 milliliter.

* Undiluted jasmine absolute may be expensive or hard to find, and in that case, you can leave it out or substitute ylang-ylang essential oil.

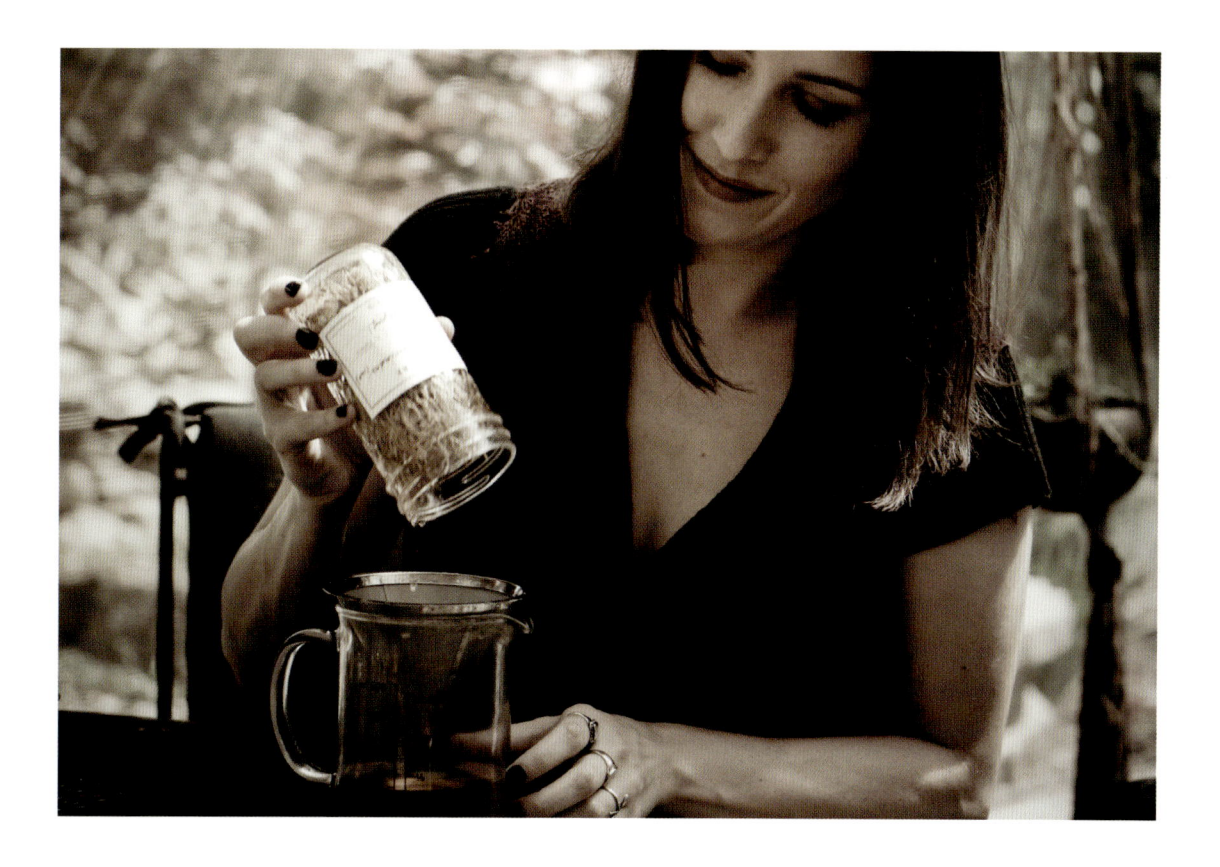

To make the kombu tincture, crush the kombu into small pieces and place it in a 4 to 8-ounce glass jar with an airtight lid. Add the botanicals, if using. Fill the jar with the alcohol, covering the kombu and botanicals completely. Allow to tincture for 3 to 4 weeks, shaking the jar occasionally. Using a fine-mesh strainer or cheesecloth, strain the liquid, discarding the solids. Reseal the tincture in the jar. Label the jar.

To make the perfume, combine the pink grapefruit, rosemary, frankincense, lavender, and bergamot essential oils and the jasmine absolute in a 1-ounce glass bottle with a fine-mist sprayer (amber or cobalt glass bottles are best). Fill the bottle to the top with the kombu tincture. Screw on the top and shake to blend. Label it and store in a cool, dark place.

What Is a Tincture?

A tincture is an infusion of a botanical material in alcohol. Usually, tinctures are made for consumption in herbalism (a milliliter or two a day used as medicine), but for most of the recipes in this book, we will be making aromatic tinctures to be used externally as perfume.

How to Tincture

Fill a glass jar three-quarters full with dried plant materials that have been cut into small pieces. (If you're using dried roots, fill the jar only halfway, as these tend to expand.)

Next, cover the plant materials with organic 190-proof alcohol, filling close to the top of the jar.

NOTE: In some tinctures, organic vodka may be used in place of higher-proof alcohol. However, tough materials like dried seeds, woods, and roots, as well as materials containing lots of water, such as fresh leaves and flowers, are better tinctured with a higher-proof alcohol. Because it is difficult to find organic alcohol with such a high proof, you may have to settle for Everclear.

Seal the jar with an airtight lid and label it with the date, the type and amount of alcohol used, and the names and amounts of botanicals used.

Shake the tincture once every few days. Depending on the density of the plant materials used and the strength of the alcohol, your tincture will need between two and six weeks of infusing time. In most cases, two weeks is sufficient, but when in doubt, let it sit longer. You can't over-tincture a tincture.

Once the extraction is finished, strain the tincture using a fine-mesh strainer or cheesecloth, discarding the plant materials.

Seal the infused alcohol in an airtight container and store it in a cool, dark place. Stored properly, your tincture will not expire.

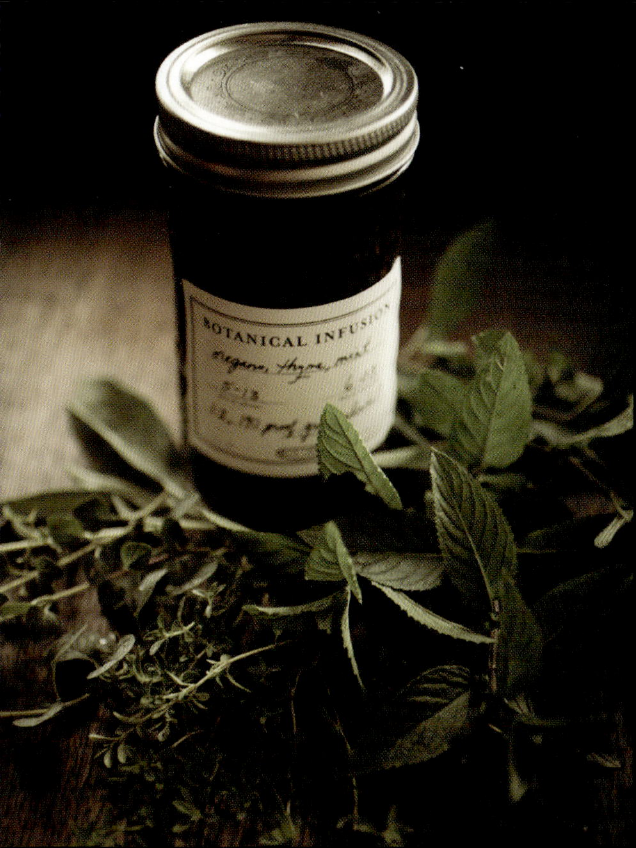
BOTANICAL INFUSION
oregano, thyme, mint
5-13
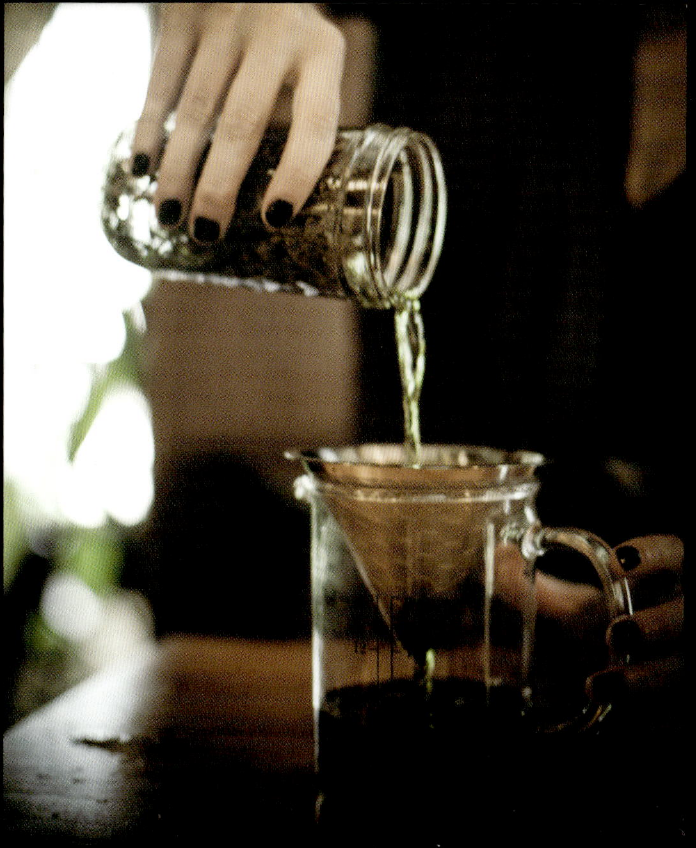
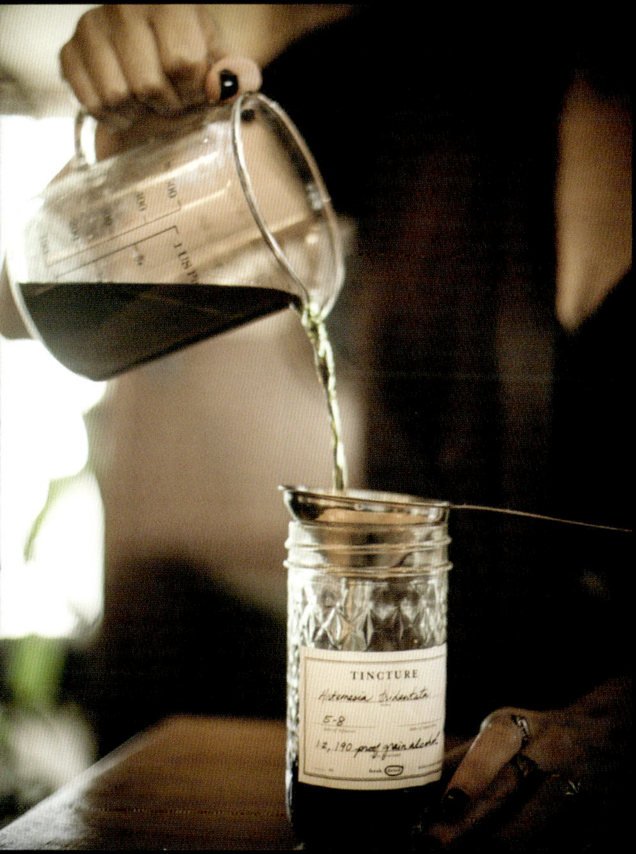
TINCTURE
Artemesia tridentata
5-8
1:2, 190 proof grain alcohol
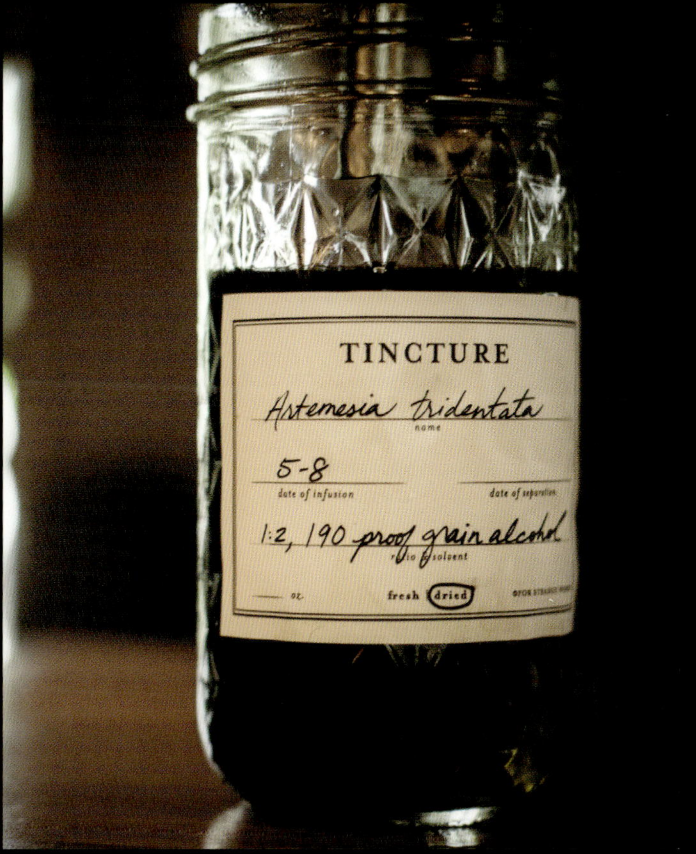
TINCTURE
Artemesia tridentata
name
5-8
date of infusion
date of separation
1:2, 190 proof grain alcohol
oz.
fresh dried

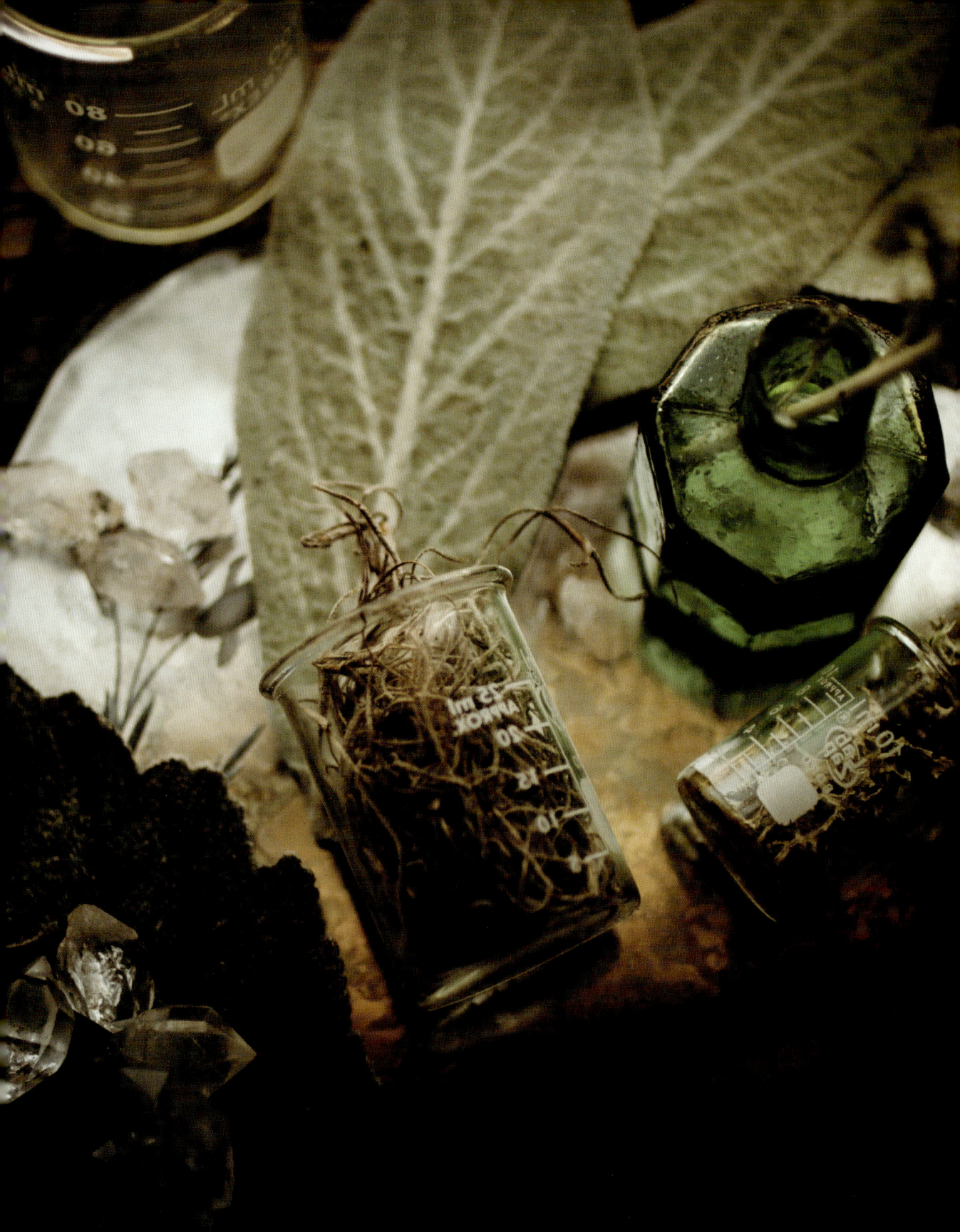

Two

ESSENTIAL OILS

Since essential oils have gained popularity in home use, many companies have begun to suggest using them as if they were whole herbs. Some websites and companies distribute this type of misinformation, including dangerous suggestions for oral consumption, because they want to sell more to consumers. **Aromatherapy is not a more convenient form of herbalism and should not be used as a substitute for herbalism.** Although some essential oils can be used as natural flavors in foods and beverages, they must be diluted and dispersed properly in order to be consumed safely. Herbalism using whole herbs is a safer, more sustainable, and more beneficial way of working with plants for most types of physical healing.

With that said, essential oils have an unparalleled, near magical ability to engage our olfactory sense. Scent molecules, interacting with the brain's hypothalamus, are able to connect us directly to our memories and emotions, creating an opportunity to remember, acknowledge, and integrate our inner landscape. A powerful form of healing, aromatherapy can impact the subconscious in ways that many other methods cannot.

A scent can help connect us to ourselves in a way that can deeply align and focus the mind on what it is truly seeking. It can create the sense of something we are craving or missing. It can enhance the aspects of our moods and personalities that we want to express and remember. It can even communicate something about us to others who come close enough.

Over the years, I've noticed that some scents attract certain personality types. For instance, **jasmine** (*Jasminum grandiflorum* or *Jasminum sambac*), also known as the "King of Flowers," is often loved most by those who wish to be seen. Perhaps they are seeking attention from the external world, or maybe they aren't receiving the attention they need in a relationship. Jasmine uplifts, energizes, and asserts its presence. Jasmine knows that those who don't stop to appreciate its blooming vine are missing out. Another example is **oakmoss** (*Evernia prunastri*). Those who are drawn to oakmoss in a perfume are likely to have a similarly grounded and earthy disposition. They are thoughtful and logical, and they may tend to be introverted and introspective. I believe this dark green lichen connects them powerfully with their intuition.

I have long kept a journal, which I often consult in order to draw connections between significant events in my life and the aromatics I was drawn to at those times. This practice has offered invaluable insight into my own healing, and it has allowed me to better address others' emotional well-being through scent. As you develop your own personal relationship with plant aromatics, I strongly encourage you to record your thoughts and feelings in response to each new interaction.

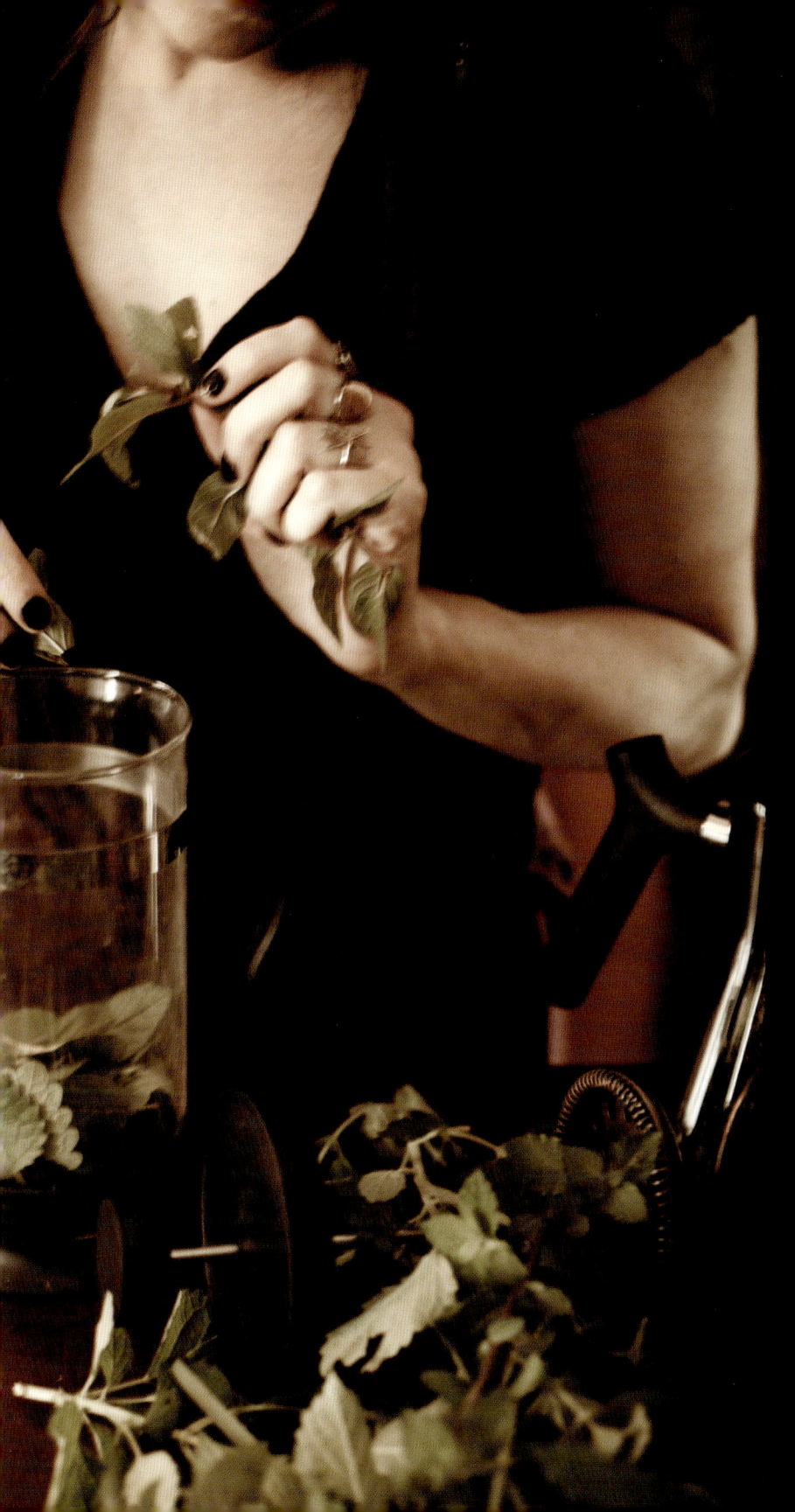

I have developed my own relationship with plants primarily through gardening and spending time outdoors. As my garden has expanded over the years, and the many beings I tend have become established, so has my relationship to the aromatics they produce. In my experience, it is most satisfying to work with an essential oil after having cultivated and cared for the plant from which it is extracted. If I work with an aromatic extract from a plant that I have not encountered, either in my garden or on hikes and travels, I make a point to study and visualize it. I think about why it produces the particular scent molecules it does, the conditions of its environment, and its adaptive responses. The scents within every leaf, resin, flower, seed, wood, bark, and root are there to relay messages. Sometimes the message is meant to intimidate invaders; other times it is meant to lure pollinators or to communicate with humans or other animals.

6. **Check the source.** The label should state which country the oil is from. Only certain essential oils, such as peppermint, lavender, lemon, orange, and cedar, are produced in the United States in large enough quantities for distribution. Most other oils are imported.

7. **Purchase in sustainable quantities.** The scent of citrus oils will begin to fade after one year, so it's best to purchase only as much as you can use in that time. Florals and the more delicate seed and herb essences will also fade or change in scent after a few years. Many of the heavier root and wood oils will actually improve with age, as will some leaf oils such as patchouli. Over time, these will become smoother and deeper.

8. **Read the ingredients.** With rare exceptions, there should be only one ingredient in the bottle, and that is the essential oil. It is sometimes acceptable, however, for expensive oils to be diluted in a carrier such as jojoba oil.

9. **If buying wild-harvested oil, consider whether it was harvested sustainably.** Wild-harvested essential oils are clean, as you can be sure they were not treated with chemicals. However, it's important to research them to be sure they were harvested ethically and sustainably. Woods are best from plantations, deadfall, and industry byproducts, as it is destructive to harvest live wild trees. If you are unsure about other materials, stick with organic (or sometimes described as "unsprayed") cultivated plants.

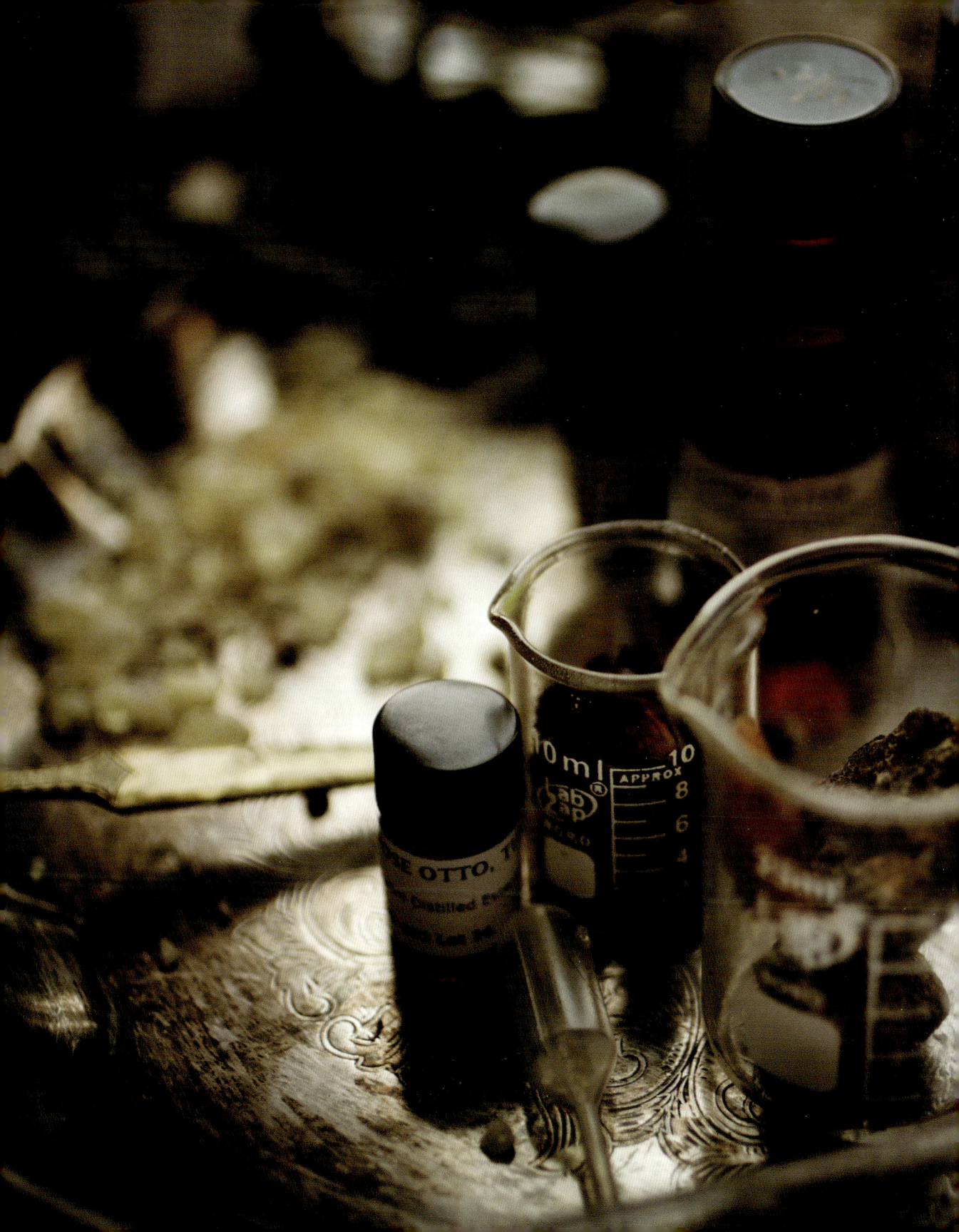

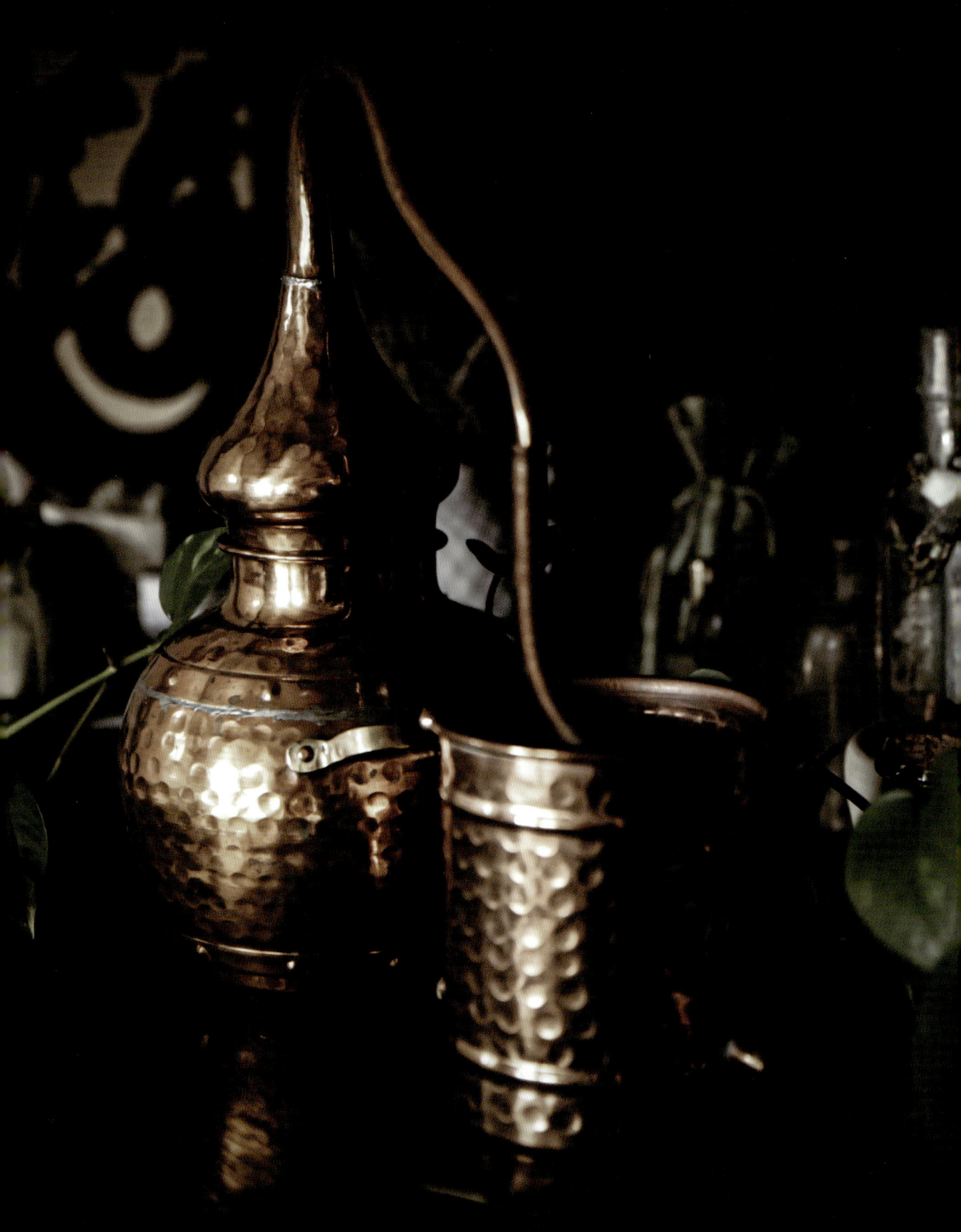

Three

BOTANICAL PERFUME

It's Not a Cosmetic

A clean diet involves more than the food we eat. Synthetic fragrances, which are found not only in perfumes but also in many candles, air "fresheners," hair products, home cleaning and laundry supplies, soaps, deodorants, and incense, are dangerous to our bodies and usually contain hormone-disrupting chemicals. They can also damage our ability to smell, overwhelming our olfactory receptors and desensitizing us to natural scents. Often, these chemicals induce headaches, and, in my opinion, they rarely smell nice. Because they are made in a lab and not in nature, their molecular components are much less complex, and the notes they produce tend to be loud and flat. Plant-based perfume is of natural origin, so it is both more complex and more nuanced.

Sadly, the commercial fragrance industry stripped perfume of its artistic and therapeutic value nearly a century ago. I use the word "strange" in my brand name in part as a way of letting customers know that I do not work within the established boundaries of this industry, where perfume is reduced to a cosmetic. Modern advertising has used fear to embed certain myths in our culture. These myths say that the purpose of perfume is to improve the wearer's sexual desirability, to shame their skin's natural scent and replace it with a chemical cocktail in a shiny bottle endorsed by a celebrity. If that is "normal," then I will gladly take on the term "strange."

I make natural perfume to provide the inner spirit a connection to nature, the mind a source of comfort or inspiration, and the body a tool for soothing or stimulating its energy. Perfume construction is also my primary creative outlet; I love experimenting with the artistic potential and aesthetic challenges plant essences present.

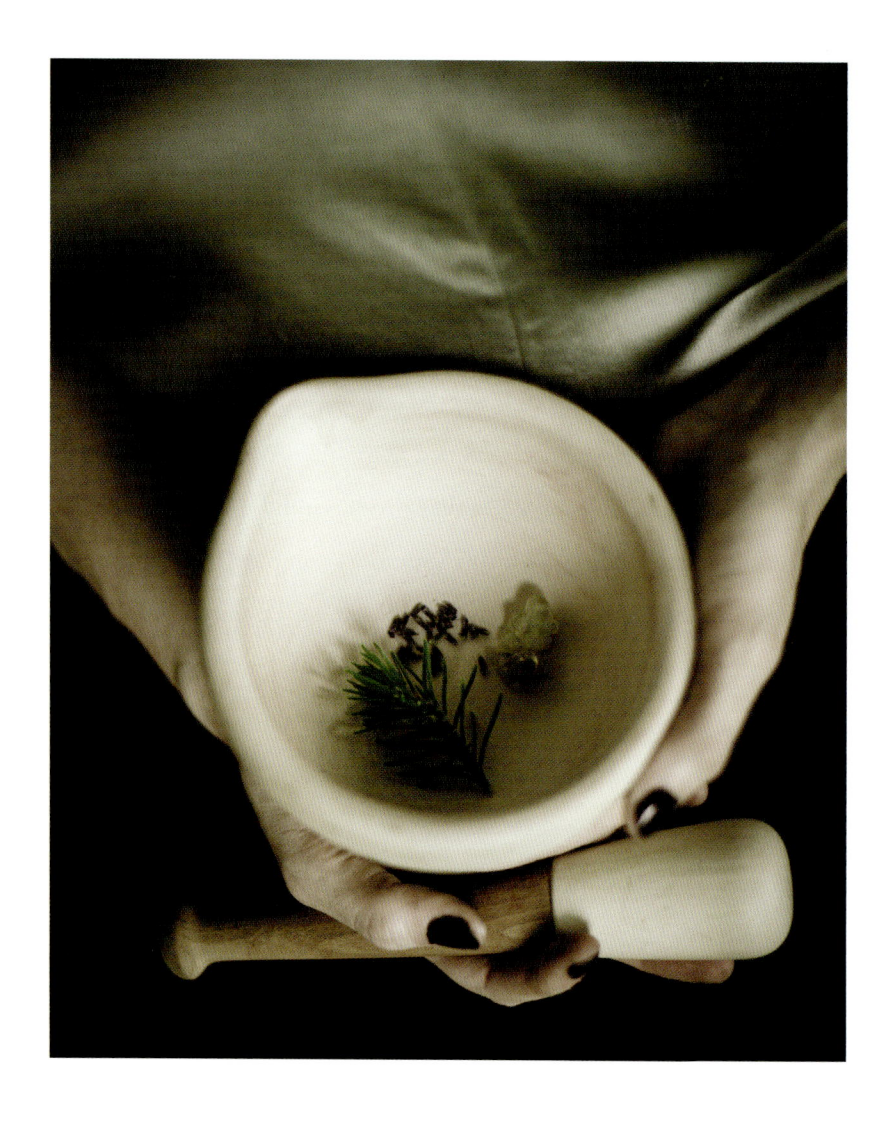

Connecting with the Senses

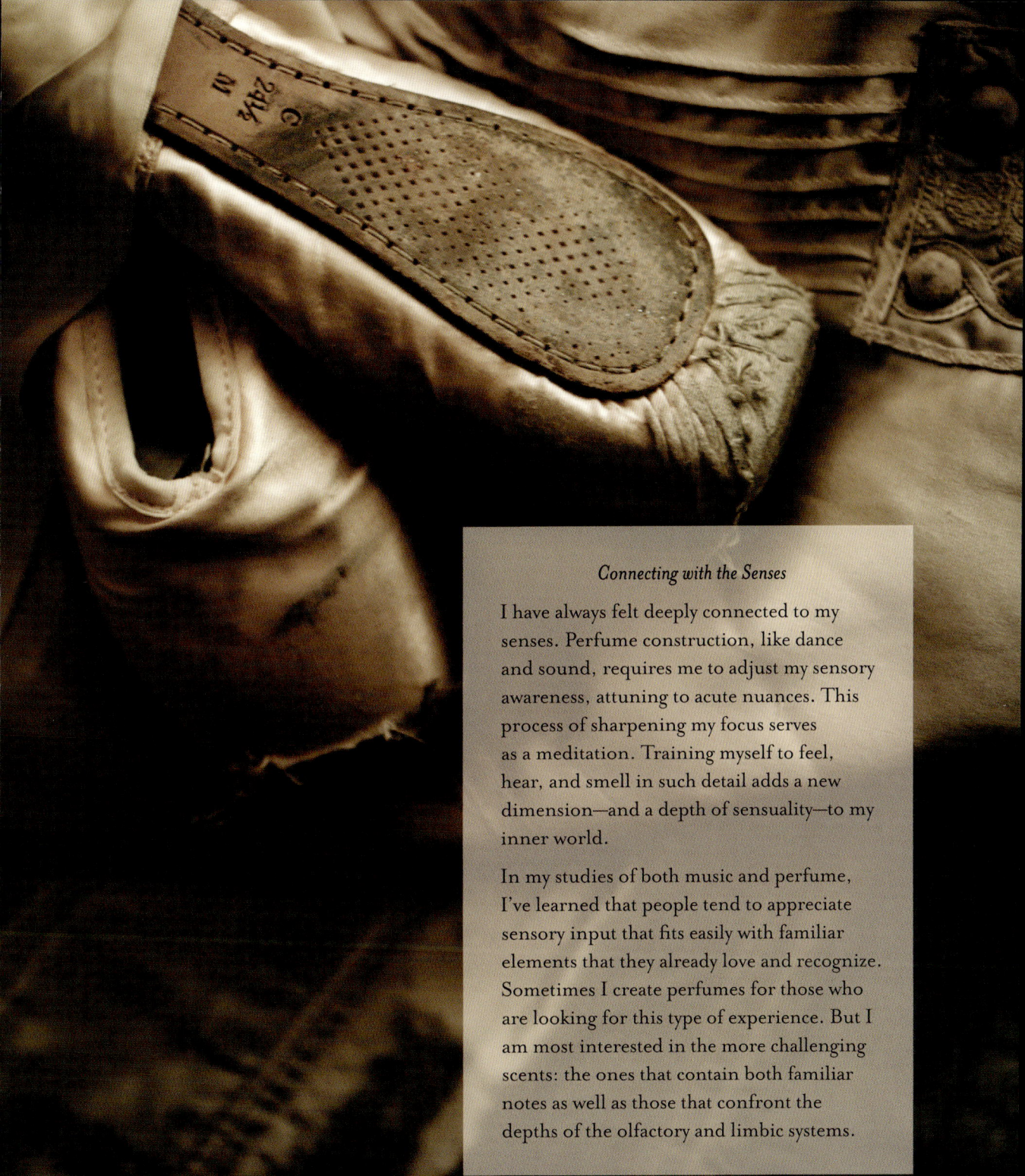

I have always felt deeply connected to my senses. Perfume construction, like dance and sound, requires me to adjust my sensory awareness, attuning to acute nuances. This process of sharpening my focus serves as a meditation. Training myself to feel, hear, and smell in such detail adds a new dimension—and a depth of sensuality—to my inner world.

In my studies of both music and perfume, I've learned that people tend to appreciate sensory input that fits easily with familiar elements that they already love and recognize. Sometimes I create perfumes for those who are looking for this type of experience. But I am most interested in the more challenging scents: the ones that contain both familiar notes as well as those that confront the depths of the olfactory and limbic systems.

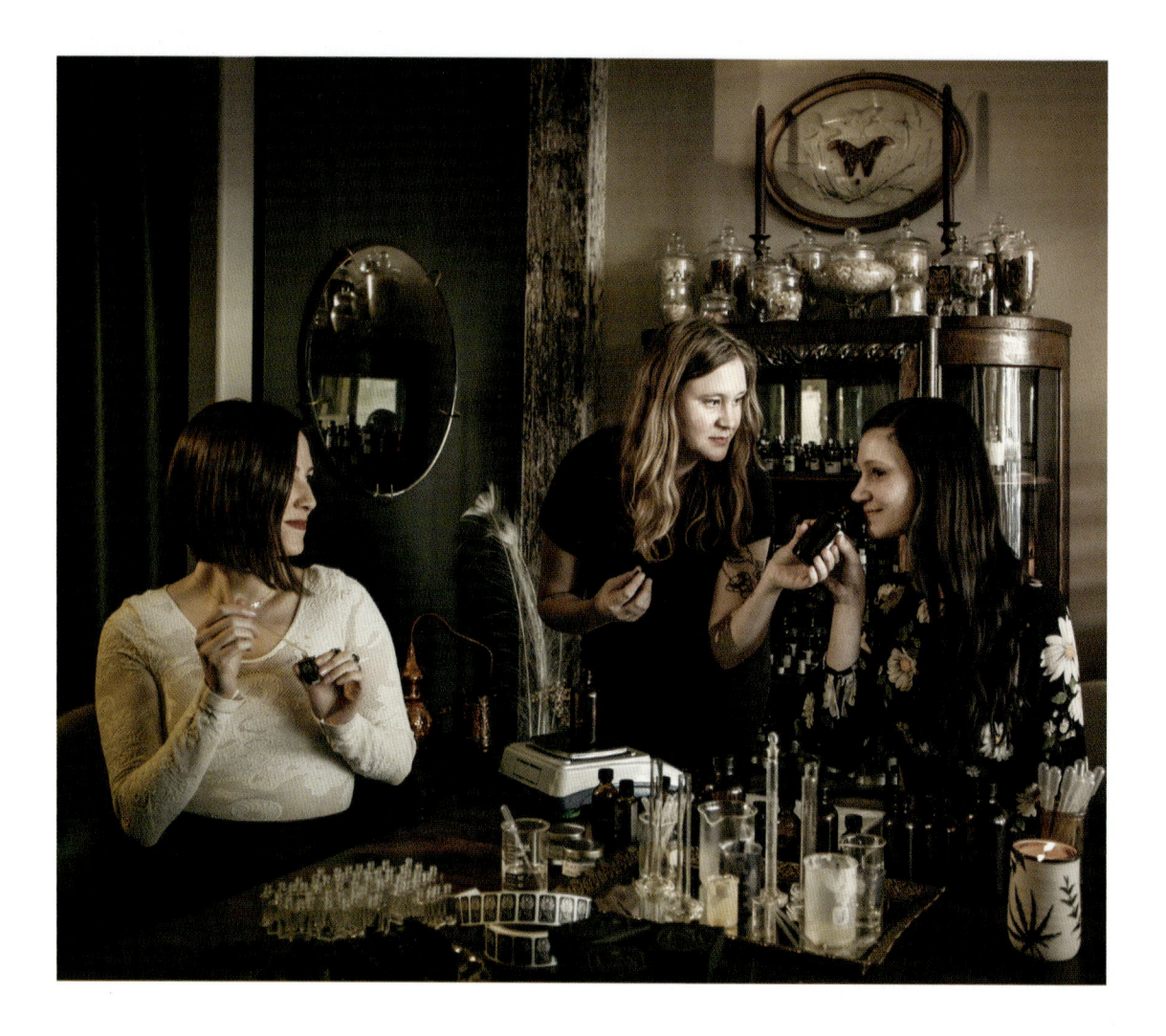

Choosing a Natural Perfume

Now that we have established that botanical perfume is not merely a tool for attracting a mate, let's focus on what it is that appeals to *you*.

To discover the natural aromatics that are best for you, take into consideration the following:

1. What does this scent remind me of?

2. Where have I smelled this before?

3. How does the scent evolve on my skin? (Record what you notice after one minute, five minutes, thirty minutes, and five hours.)

4. Compared with how it smells on a neutral test strip, how is the scent affected by my skin? Does my skin tend to turn the scent sweeter? More sour? Smokier? Spicier?

5. What aromatherapy effects am I looking for in a perfume? Do I want to balance my temperament with an opposing frequency or match my mood with a similar frequency?

6. Why am I attracted to these notes? Does wood oil make me feel stronger? Do resinous notes make me feel comforted? Do flowers make me feel softer or more feminine? Do I have an affinity for certain plants in my life that energetically resonate with me?

7. What natural scents have I experienced that connect me to scent memories of other times in my life, and which seem to be associated with the most positive emotions? (Examples: the place you grew up, childhood toys, camping, gardening, books, Grandma's house, open markets, farm and country, mountains, candy or beverages, travels, cooking scents, church, someone who was close to you.)

Production of Botanical Perfume

Producing natural perfume is typically expensive and labor intensive. Plant essences are delicate and require specific storage conditions, and their supply is variable, unlike synthetics. For these reasons, it's difficult to produce natural perfumes in large quantities while maintaining consistency among batches. The art of botanical perfume production remains in the hands of several small, independent businesses whose proprietors have dedicated themselves to the challenges of working within the natural realm.

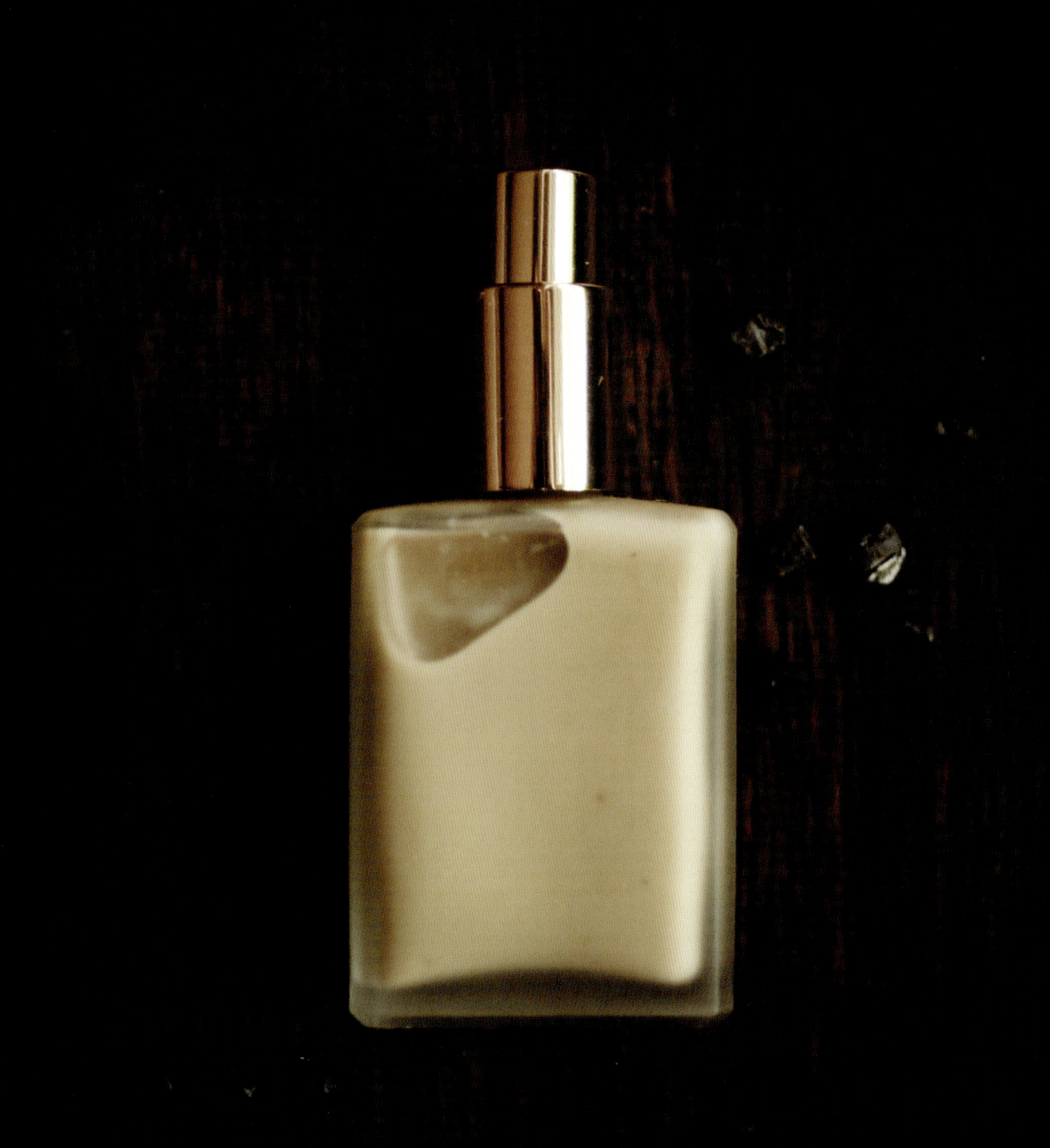

Four

SYNESTHESIA

There are some aspects of working with scent that, for me, are best understood through synesthesia. Long before I began For Strange Women, I was involved in music. I played violin, wrote songs in bands, and studied music production and recording in college.

When I began working with aromatics, I realized that mixing scent was very similar to mixing sound. Just as a perfumer works with multiple elements to produce a full-bodied scent, a sound engineer's job is to render many layers of sound into a clear and balanced mix. Sometimes you have two instruments creating sounds in the same frequency range, and when this happens, one will "bury" the other since they are competing for the same space. Replace "instruments" with "essences" and "sounds" with "scents," and you have a common scenario in my perfume studio.

The concept of using sound vocabulary to describe scent is nothing new. Perfume construction is often referred to in terms of "notes" within a chord (base note, middle note, and top note). While this can be helpful, many of my perfumes contain over twenty essences—or twenty "notes"—and a musical chord of this complexity would sound like a mess. For this reason, I've found the tools and vocabulary of audio engineering to be a better fit. The shift from music to perfume was an unexpected one for me, but a natural progression at the same time. The following are some of the concepts from my sound-mixing days that I now apply to my work with perfume.

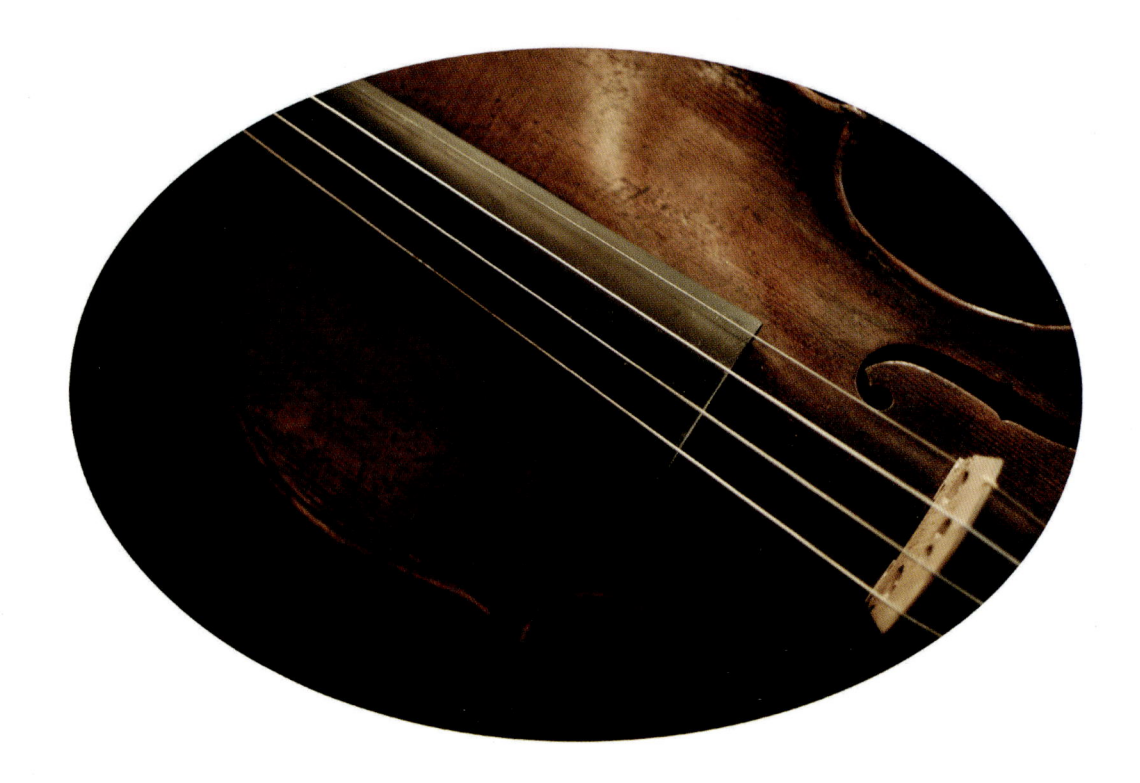

REVERBERATION (RESONANCE)

The size of the room and the hardness of the surfaces in it affect the type and amount of reverberation. This can be artificially added to recordings and live effects, and it can also be naturally heard in live performances. It creates a sense of how large a space is and how far away you are from the source of the sound. That's how the brain gives you depth perception beyond your eyes. It creates a sense of expansion and depth from the reflected layers. It also makes the tonality a bit more forgiving as the reflections smooth out imperfections and give the impression that the instrument is farther away, behind other instruments. *Reverberation (or resonance) can be detected in scents that are syrupy and resinous, sweet and expansive. Resonance enhances sillage and creates depth while adding sweetness that smooths over less-forgiving elements.*

EQUALIZATION

The equalization can be shaped for each recorded track to cut back on certain recorded frequencies and enhance other areas of the frequency. This creates "pockets" for separate voices and instruments to exist within so that they are not competing with one another. This technique preserves clarity. *An aromatic example: Patchouli and geranium share some of the same frequency range, so mixing the two will have a muddying effect. Since scent equalization cannot be manipulated digitally, it is best, when two scents are competing with one another, to go with a different combination of essences.*

WAVEFORMS

The timbre of a sound depends on the shape of the waveform produced. Simply put, waveforms can contain sharp, harsh edges or softer, rounded edges. Sharper waveforms (saw waves) will stand out more in a mix, while the softer waveforms (sine waves) will sound the most pleasing and blend the most easily. *Think of black peppercorn as a saw wave and rose as a sine wave. The texture of any composition is much more interesting when it includes a combination of waveforms that create soft as well as more structured shapes.*

ATTACK

The "attack" describes how quickly a sound reaches its full volume. *Some notes reach our olfactory system quickly, while others emerge later as the blend evolves on the skin. "Top notes" are typically scents with a fast attack, as their molecules are the smallest and most volatile. "Base notes" are known for their slow attack; they sometimes go undetected on the skin for hours before reaching their full volume.*

--- **RELEASE** ---

The "release" describes how long a sound takes to fade after the attack. *Also called the "dry down" of each essence in a blend, a scent's release may be long or short. Often, a perfume is most interesting when the essences it contains have a variety of release times. This effect is usually only detectable in natural perfumes, as synthetic scents tend to have a blunt attack and release of the entire composition.*

--- **CHORUS** ---

This modulation splits a single voice into several, slightly different voices. Everyone's voice has its own timbre, volume, pitch, etc. Creating layers of sound with slight variation in these qualities adds chorus depth. *In the same way, I use plant essences to compose chorus effects in a perfume. For example, two different varieties of basil are singing the same song. But when they sing the song in unison, their voices sound stronger and fuller, because one variety is sweeter and the other is darker and spicier. Several tree resins can be used to create a resin chorus, or several woods to create a wood chorus.*

Here is a visual map of a simple perfume as it exists in my mind when I create it. This is similar to how my mind would organize a map of instrument tracks when I used to record music. Synesthesia has allowed those soundscapes to become "scentscapes."

H
I
G
H

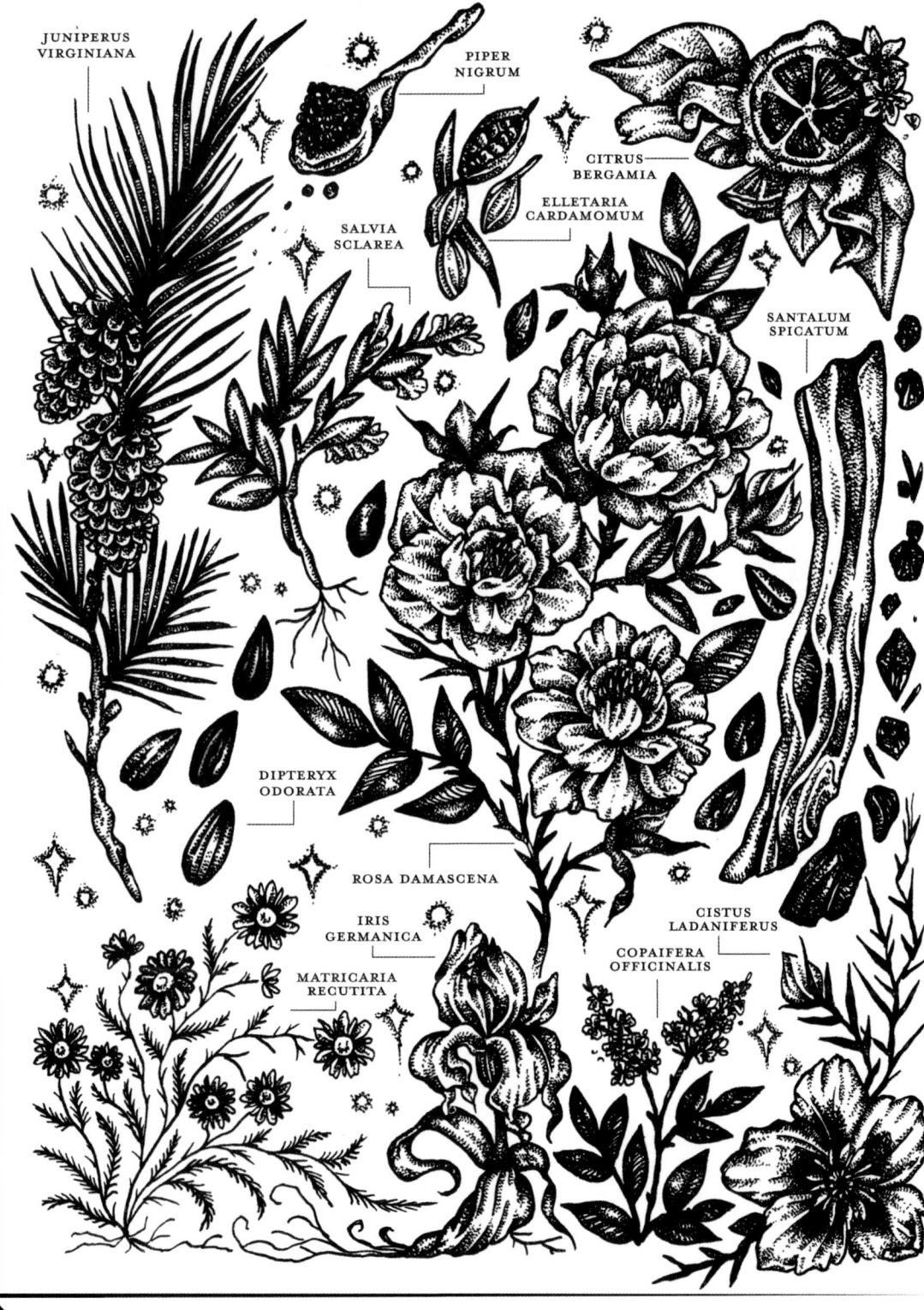

F
R
E
Q
U
E
N
C
Y

L
O
W

JUNIPERUS
VIRGINIANA

PIPER
NIGRUM

CITRUS
BERGAMIA

SALVIA
SCLAREA

ELLETARIA
CARDAMOMUM

SANTALUM
SPICATUM

DIPTERYX
ODORATA

ROSA DAMASCENA

IRIS
GERMANICA

CISTUS
LADANIFERUS

MATRICARIA
RECUTITA

COPAIFERA
OFFICINALIS

DRY —to— RESINOUS

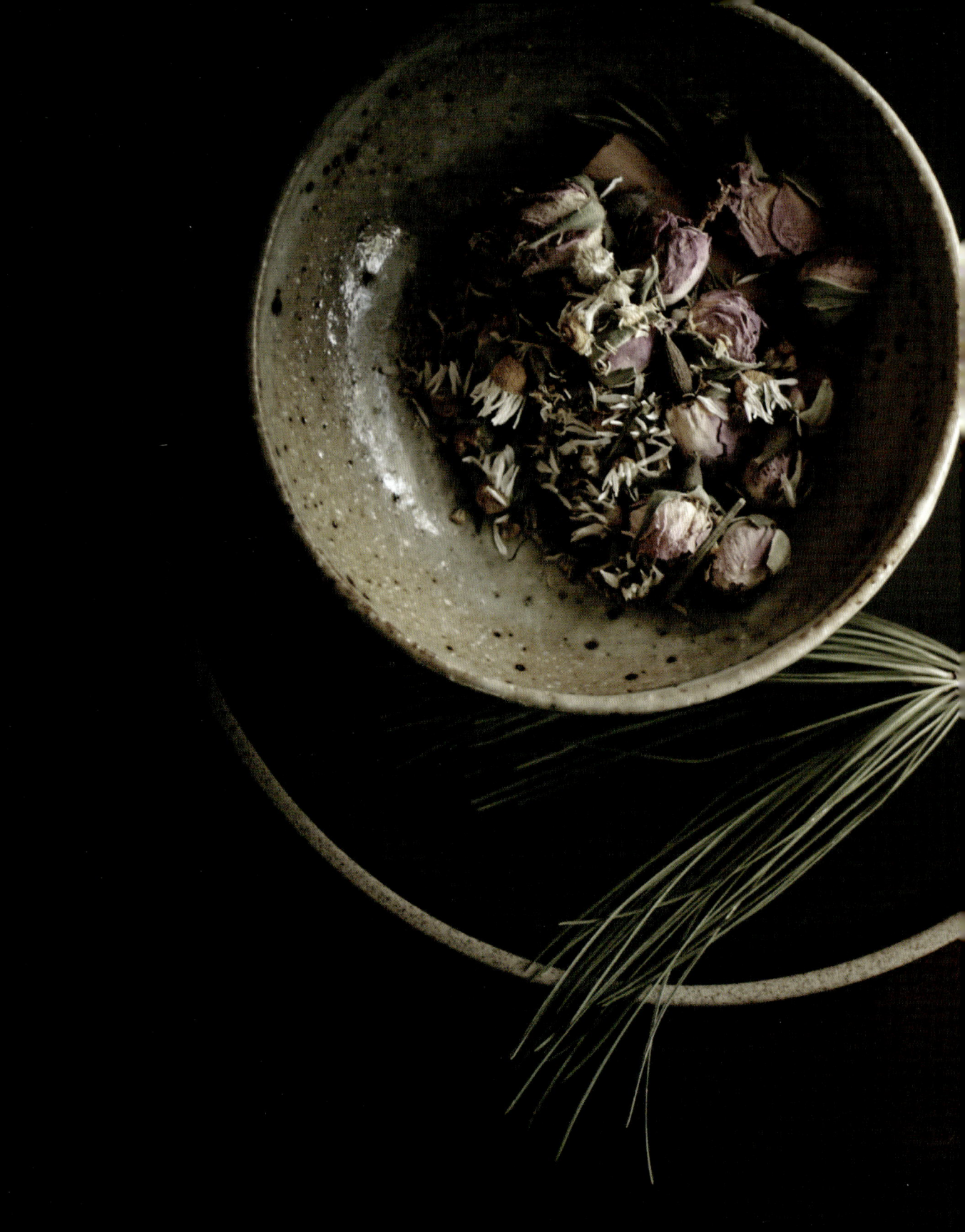

Five

BOTANICAL MATERIALS

Citrus oils are known for their ability to energize and uplift. They are antidepressants. Certain citrus oils, like grapefruit, bergamot, and orange, are able to pull us out of a dark mood instantly. The relief is temporary, but it can be just enough to set us back in motion when we have lost momentum. The essential oils of citrus, pressed from the outer rind, are inexpensive and relatively abundant since most are by-products of the fruit industry. However, these essential oils can be photosensitizing when applied to the skin if they are not properly diluted, and even then, it's important to limit sun exposure if wearing citrus.

Seeds contain the potential—the DNA—of the plant. Their scent can be sweet or savory, and upon drying, the scents (and flavors) often intensify, unlike many flowers and leaves, which tend to lose their scent after drying. I find seeds to have uplifting, inspirational qualities. They stimulate the mind and connect me with the possibilities of my own potential. Seeds must be nurtured and encouraged to develop, and I believe they contain that same nurturing energy. When I introduce someone to single essences, the seed oils usually induce feelings of certainty, confidence, and positivity.

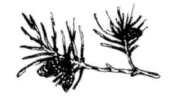

CARDAMOM AND SPRUCE TEA

Serves 1

1 2-inch fresh cut of spruce needles (easy to wild-harvest in many regions)

2 cardamom pods

Using a mortar and pestle, crush the spruce needles and cardamom pods. Add the crushed ingredients to a cup of boiled filtered water, infusing for 10 minutes. Pour the tea through a tea strainer or gaiwan tea set, pictured; discard the solids.

CARDAMOM SEED

(*Elettaria cardamomum*) Cardamom was highly prized in ancient Persian, Arabian, and Indian cultures for its antidepressant, aphrodisiac, and energizing qualities. Often used as a culinary ingredient, it also lends itself beautifully to perfume, blending well with woods, resins, evergreen needles, and other spices. Cardamom is known to be a powerful antioxidant and digestive stimulant. When using cardamom in the kitchen, always purchase the freshest green pods available and store them away from sunlight. Crush the seeds with a mortar and pestle (or *suribachi*) right before using them; never buy ground seeds, as they lose their potency quickly.

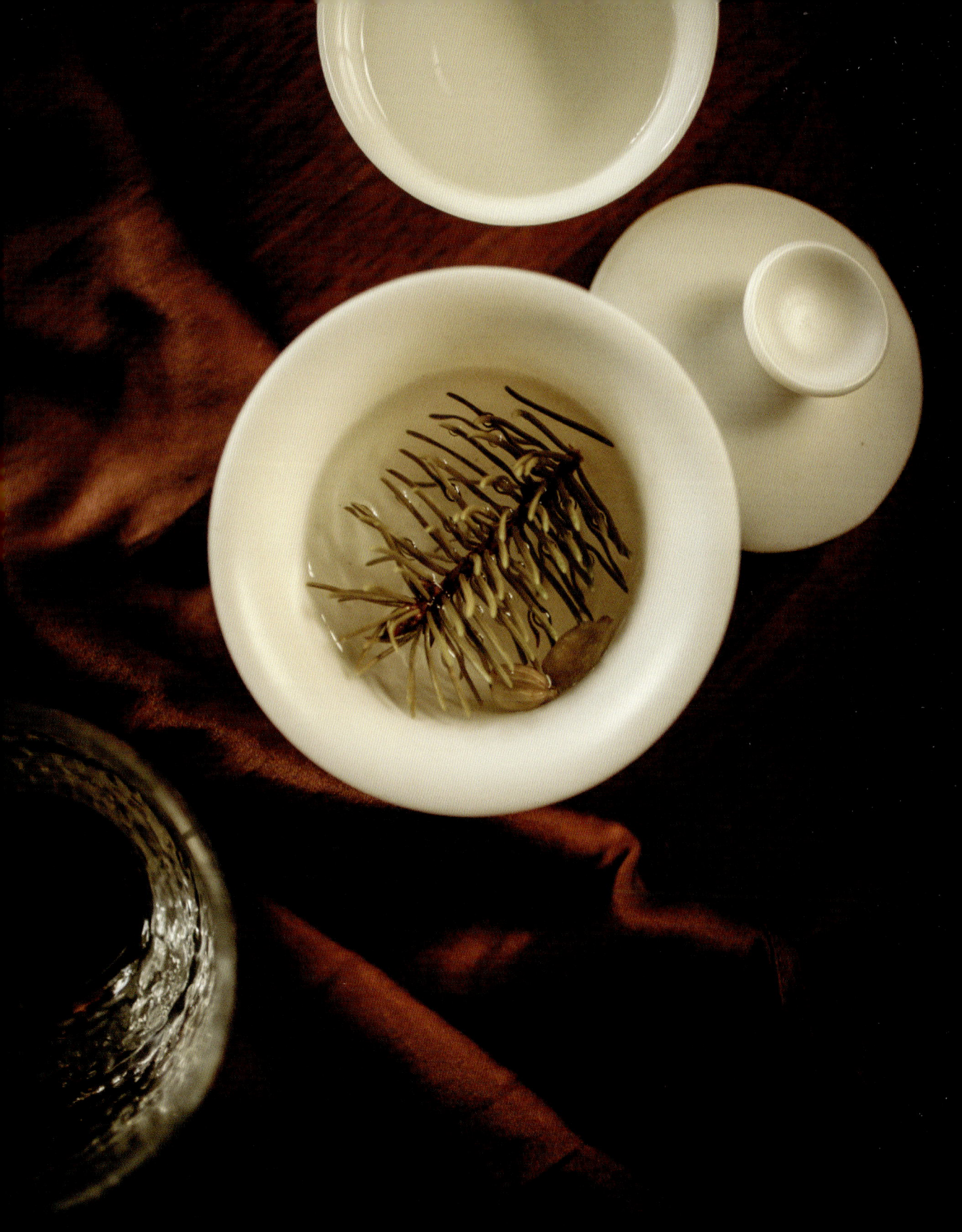

VANILLA

(*Vanilla planifolia*) In 2017, Madagascar was hit by Hurricane Enawo, creating a worldwide shortage of vanilla. At the time of this writing, Madagascar is still struggling to recover from this disaster and has received little support. Before the cost of vanilla skyrocketed due to the shortage, many took it for granted as a perfume and culinary ingredient. While its reputation in our culture is one of convention and mundanity, natural vanilla is truly a treasure, and my most loved perfumes contained a significant amount of it before the hurricane. Vanilla has the ability to soften and disperse any other ingredient, rounding out sharp edges and creating a sense of comfort. Perhaps this is why we often include it in our baked goods and home scents.

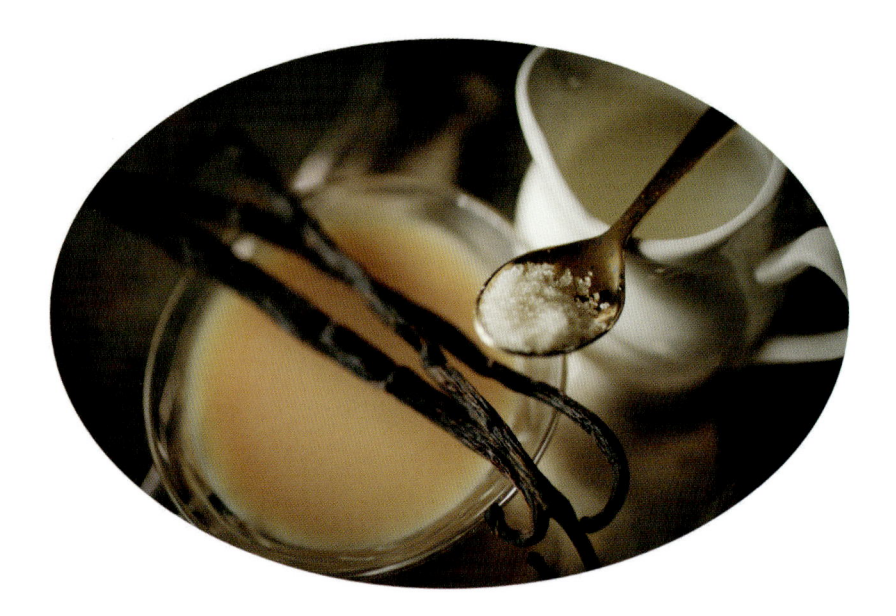

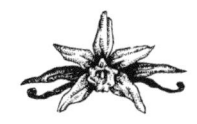

LONDON FOG LIP BALM

Makes 3 ounces by weight

NOTE: For this recipe, you will need either three 1-ounce jars/tins, six ½-ounce jars/tins, or about 20 lip balm tubes.

I find lip balm to be a convenient vehicle for aromatherapy. It can be lightly "flavored" by combining essential oils and infused oils with a sweetener, and since the balm is applied close to the nose, only a very small amount of scent is needed.

London Fog is a classic Earl Grey tea latte, sweetened with vanilla and honey. It is one of my favorite scent combinations. Sadly, I have had to discontinue my perfume inspired by it due to the vanilla shortage. Instead, I recommend this lip balm recipe, which requires much less vanilla.

1½ tablespoons loose black tea (Earl Grey is best)
¼ teaspoon vanilla powder (seeds)
½ teaspoon 190-proof alcohol
1½ ounces sweet almond oil (or avocado oil)
½ ounce (by weight) grated beeswax
1 ounce (by weight) shea butter
1 teaspoon raw creamed honey or 10 drops stevia extract
10 drops bergapten-free bergamot essential oil

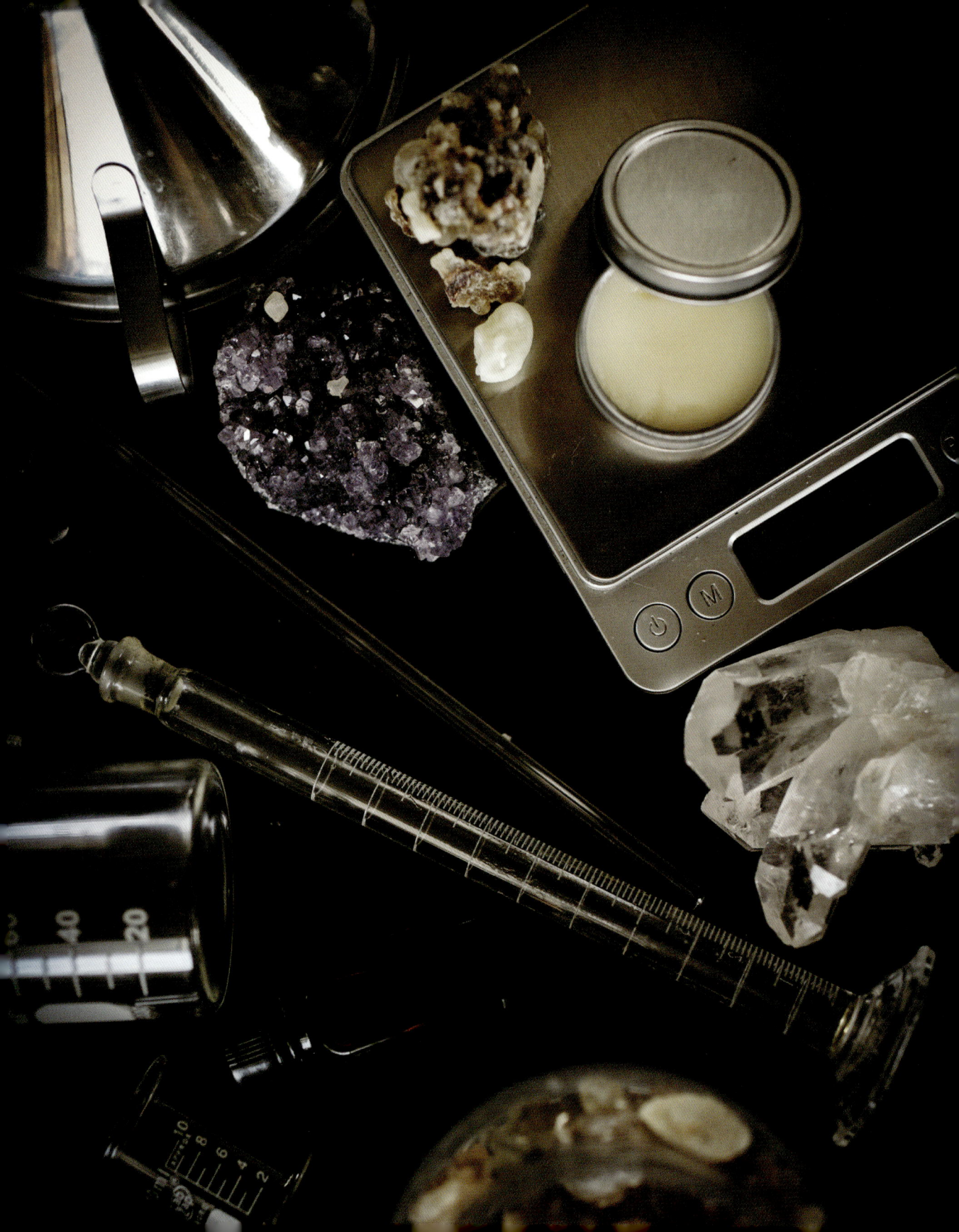

Grind the black tea using a mortar and pestle and combine with the vanilla powder in a container. Add the alcohol to the mixture and stir. Heat the almond oil in a double boiler on the stove to 200°F or in a heat-safe measuring cup in the microwave for about 1 minute. Pour the hot oil into the container with the tea and stir. The alcohol will evaporate. Allow to infuse for at least 1 hour.

Strain the oil infusion through a fine-mesh strainer or cheesecloth, pressing out the oil into a bowl and discarding the tea. It's OK to have fine tea and vanilla particles left in the oil.

Combine and melt the beeswax and shea butter in a double boiler on the stove or in a heat-safe measuring cup in the microwave. Stir occasionally and remove immediately from the heat when fully melted.

Add the tea-infused oil to the beeswax and shea butter combination, returning to the heat if the mixture begins to solidify. Stir until combined. Add the honey while the mixture is still hot, stirring thoroughly.

After the mixture begins to cool (but before it solidifies), add the bergamot essential oil. Stir. Pour into the lip balm containers of your choice and let cool. Store sealed in a cool, dark place.

Flowers are communicators. They are filled with signals that are designed to send messages to pollinators and interact with our sensory nervous system, even from a long distance away. And because of their visual and olfactory beauty, they easily capture our attention.

ROSE

(*Rosa damascena*) Rose is my favorite floral aromatic for relieving physical stress. It is known to reduce cortisol (the stress hormone), and the scent invites us to slow down to fully interpret its complexity. Rose Otto, the essential oil, is very expensive because it requires about sixty roses to produce a single drop of oil. However, the by-product of essential oil production is a distilled water called a **hydrosol**. A large amount of this water imprinted with traces of essential oil is created in every distilled batch.

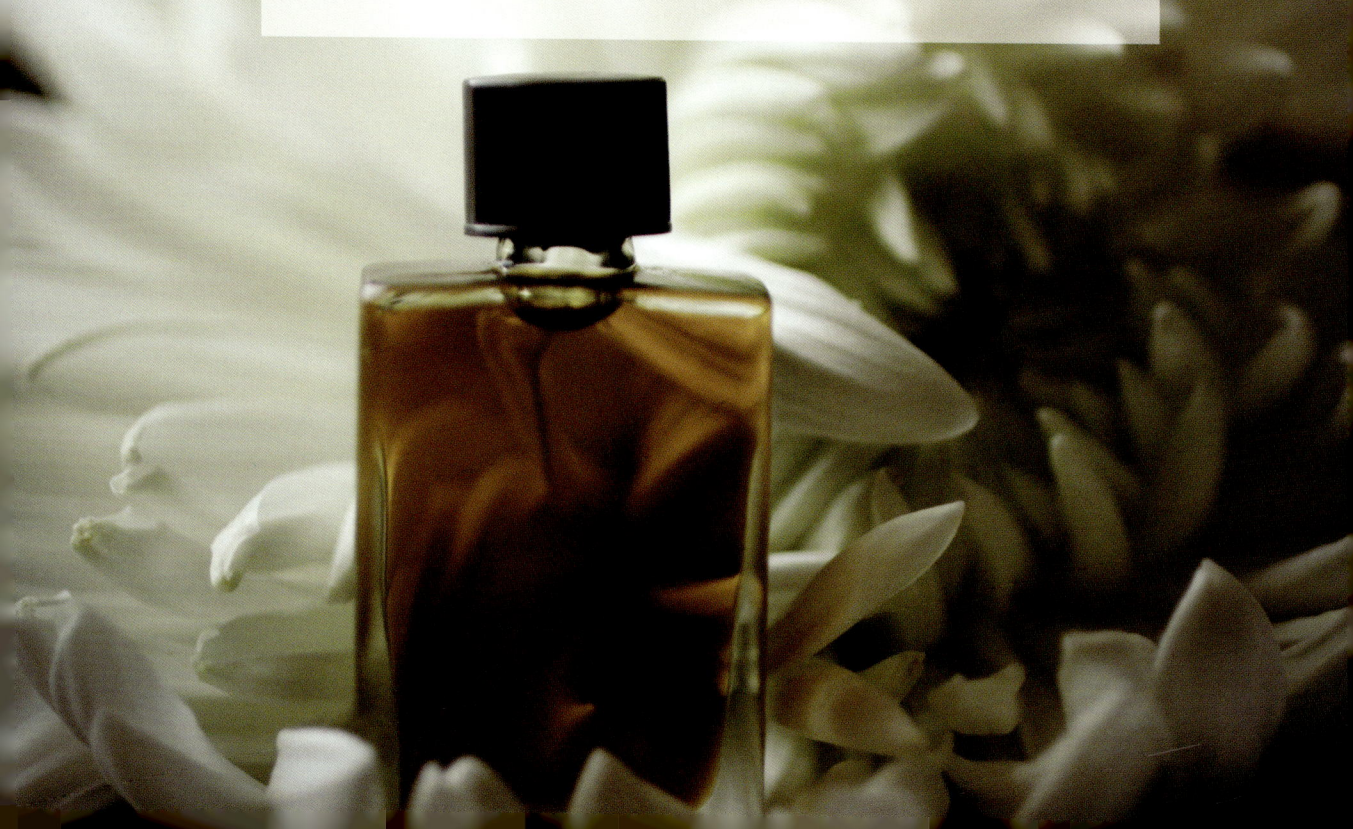

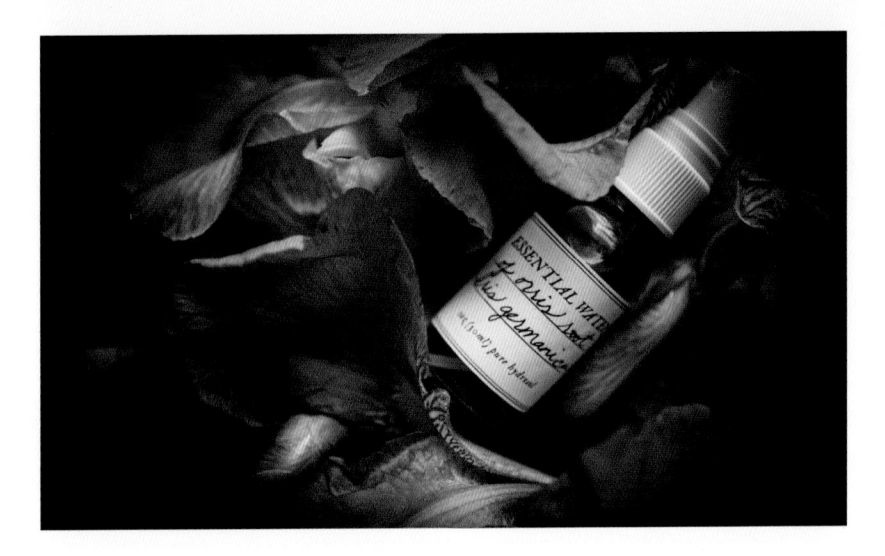

A Note on Hydrosols

In most essential oil production, the hydrosol is thrown out because it is difficult to protect from bacterial growth, but waters such as rose and orange blossom are so precious that they are often kept sterile or preserved for culinary use. As the world of aromatherapy expands, expect more availability of these distilled waters, as they are so much more abundant and sustainable for everyday use than essential oils. Only trace amounts of the plant essences are necessary for healing benefits, and because hydrosols have such a small amount of the plant's essence trapped within them, it is safe to use them to flavor food and drinks and even to use them on the face as a skin toner.

True hydrosols are clear, not colored. They are typically sold in clear glass bottles and stored in a refrigerator to prevent bacterial growth, and they must be used within eight to ten months of production. Keep in mind that markets often sell "rose water" or "orange blossom water" that has added colors, preservatives, and artificial flavor. Many of these waters are completely artificial and are not usable. Health food stores have begun to carry real hydrosols with a bit of added preservative, and while this type of formulation is good for external use, be sure to check if it is food safe. Until there is more demand for store distribution, it may be easiest to find pure hydrosol suppliers online.

At home, one of my favorite rituals is to make experimental floral lemonades. They are easy to make, they replenish minerals, and the floral notes they contain create the sense of sipping a hypnotic bouquet. I serve them in wineglasses so that their scent is enhanced by the shape of the glass.

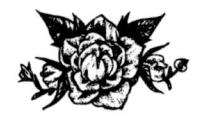

ROSE WATER LEMONADE

Serves 1

8 ounces sparkling mineral water, chilled

1 tablespoon lemon juice (approximately half a lemon)

6 drops stevia extract

1 teaspoon rose water (organic rose hydrosol)

Combine all of the ingredients in a glass and serve chilled.

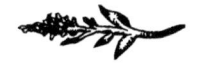

LAVENDER LEMONADE

Serves 1

8 ounces sparkling mineral water, chilled

1 tablespoon lemon juice (approximately half a lemon)

6 drops stevia extract

12 drops lavender tincture*

*The lavender tincture (see page 49) needs to be prepared two weeks in advance.

Combine all of the ingredients in a glass and serve chilled. Reserve any remaining tincture for another use.

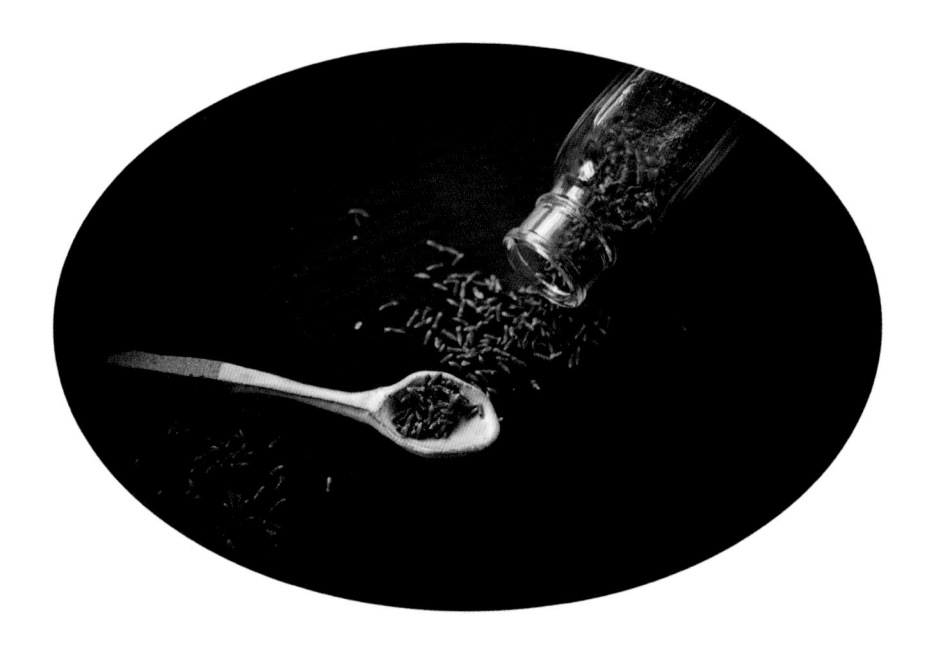

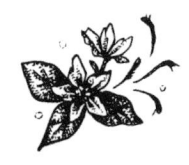

SAFFRON AND ORANGE BLOSSOM LEMONADE

Serves 1

5 saffron stamens

1 tablespoon lemon juice (approximately half a lemon)

8 ounces sparkling mineral water, chilled

6 drops stevia extract

½ teaspoon orange blossom water (neroli hydrosol)

Add the saffron to the lemon juice. Allow to infuse for 15 minutes. Combine the infused lemon juice with the other ingredients in a glass and serve chilled.

Leaves typically have a bright, crisp aromatic profile that protects the plant from pests. We find these herbal scents to be relaxing and clean, and incorporating them into our homes, food, and perfume can create the feeling of a fresh start. The ability of these scents to gently focus the mind also makes them perfect for meditation work.

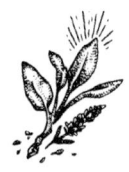

LAVENDER AND SAGE TEA

Serves 1 to 2

2 to 3 fresh common sage leaves

5 to 7 lavender buds

Small piece of frankincense resin (optional)

Raw unfiltered honey (optional)

Combine the sage and lavender in boiled filtered water and let steep for 5 minutes in a small tea cup or gaiwan tea set. Strain out the sage and lavender. For more complexity, add the frankincense and honey.

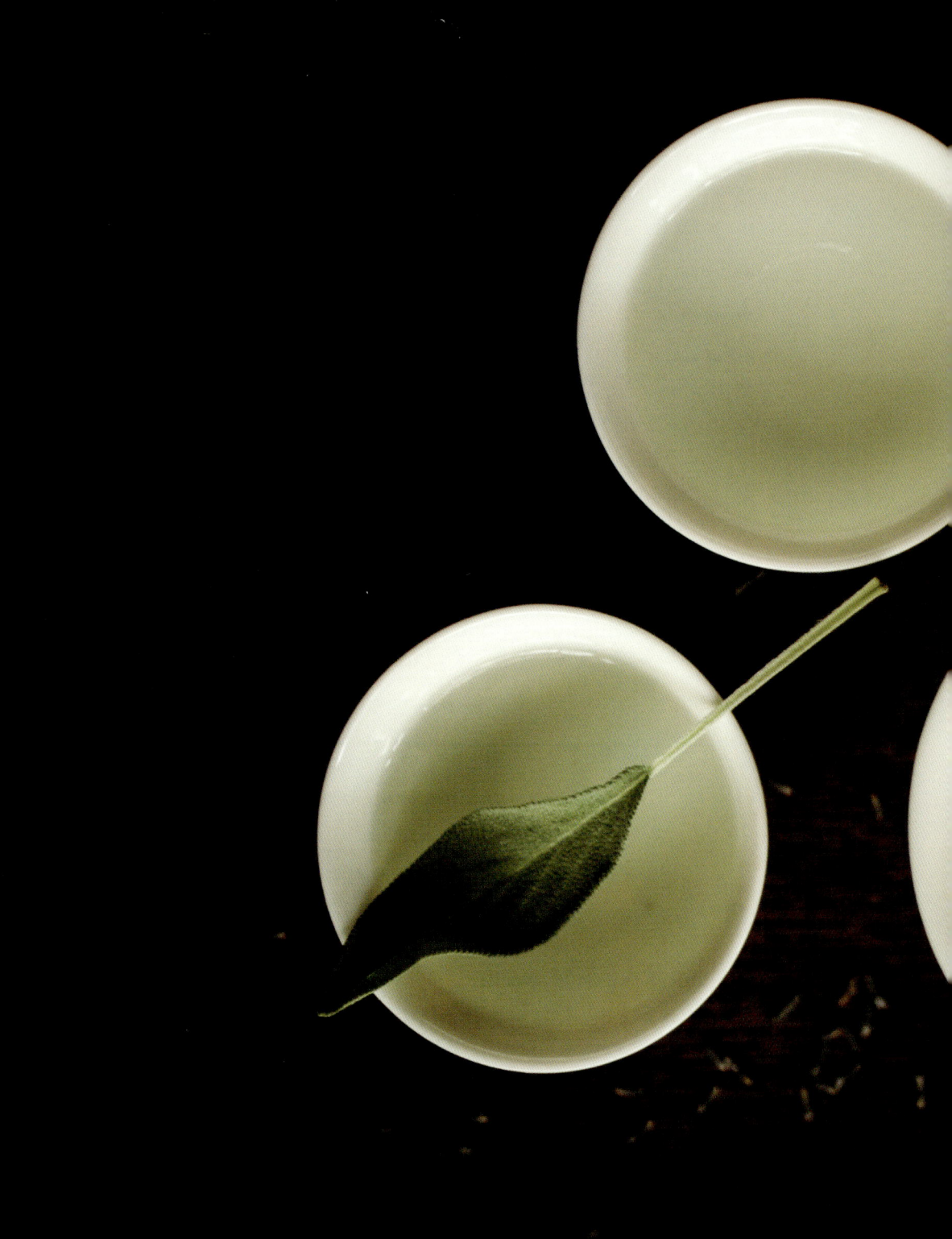

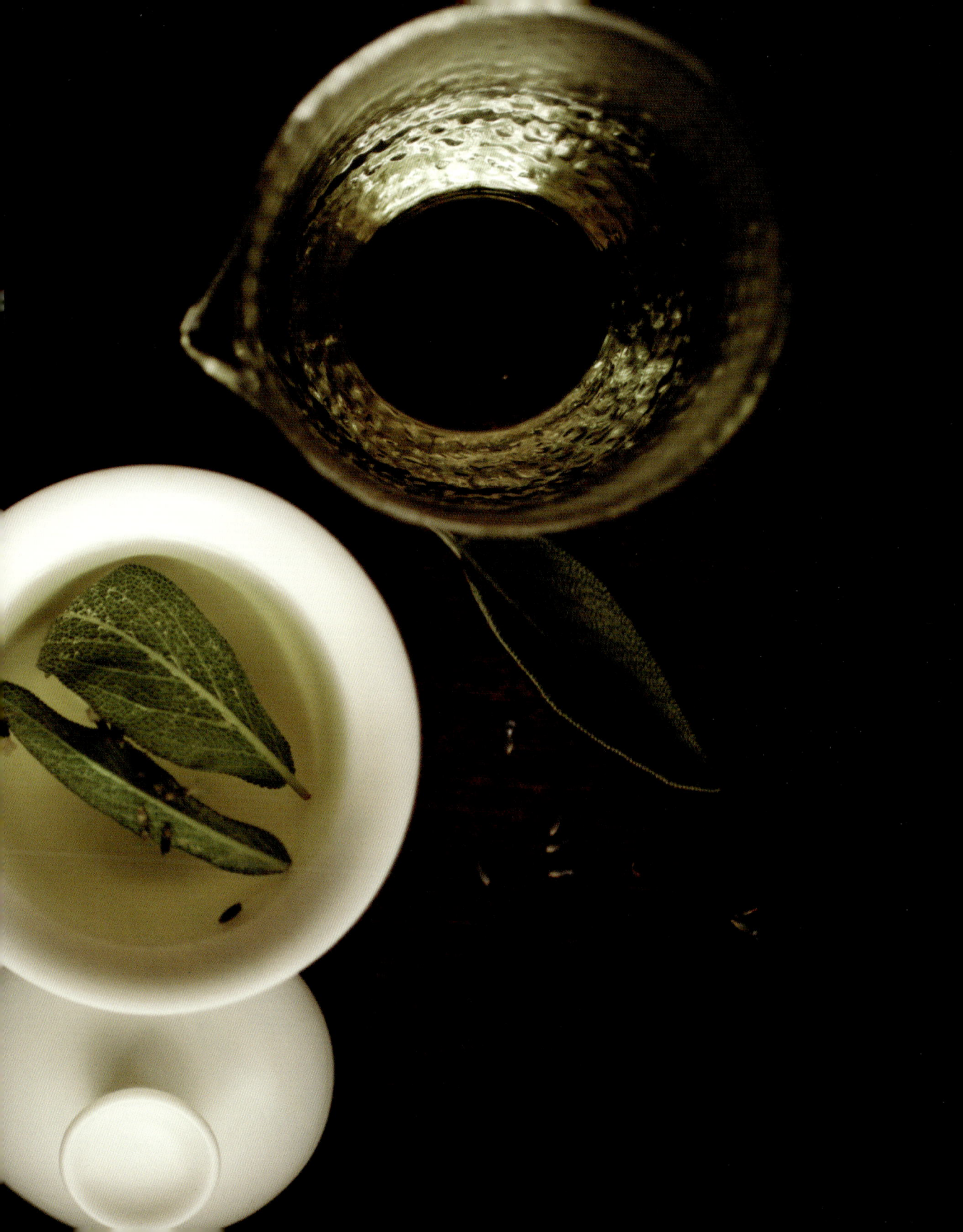

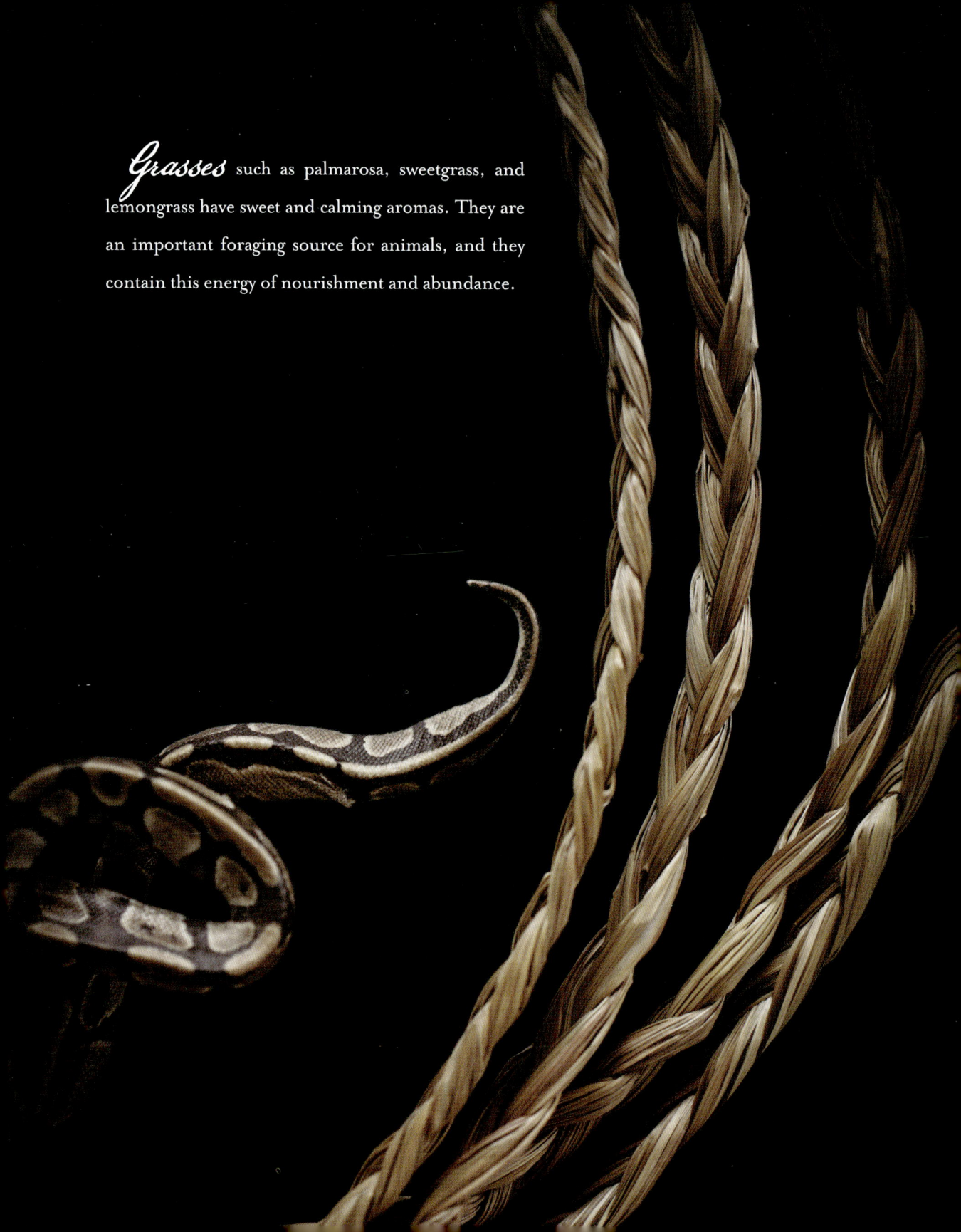

Grasses such as palmarosa, sweetgrass, and lemongrass have sweet and calming aromas. They are an important foraging source for animals, and they contain this energy of nourishment and abundance.

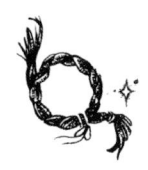

CALMING PERFUME MIST: A ROOM, BODY, OR LINEN SPRAY

Makes 1 ounce

This perfumed mist includes a soothing tincture of dried sweetgrass, which is one of my favorite materials to tincture for room and linen sprays. As the grass dries, it becomes rich in coumarin, which has the warm scent of alfalfa, hay, and vanilla.

SWEETGRASS TINCTURE

¼ cup dried sweetgrass, cut into 1-inch pieces

Organic vodka or organic 190-proof alcohol

LAVENDER TINCTURE

¼ cup organic fresh or dried lavender buds

Organic vodka or organic 190-proof alcohol

MIST

15 milliliters sweetgrass tincture

15 milliliters lavender tincture

6 drops ylang-ylang essential oil

12 drops clary sage essential oil

To make the sweetgrass tincture, place the sweetgrass in an 8-ounce jar with an airtight lid and pour in enough vodka to cover the sweetgrass completely. Seal and allow to infuse for 2 weeks, shaking occasionally. Pour the tincture through a fine-mesh strainer or cheesecloth; discard the sweetgrass. Seal and label the jar, storing away from heat and sunlight.

To make the lavender tincture, place the lavender buds in an 8-ounce jar with an airtight lid and pour in enough vodka to cover the lavender completely. Seal and allow to infuse for 2 weeks, shaking occasionally. Pour the tincture through a fine-mesh strainer or cheesecloth; discard the lavender. Seal and label the jar, storing away from heat and sunlight.

To make the mist, combine 15 milliliters of sweetgrass tincture and 15 milliliters of lavender tincture in a small glass liquid measuring cup or beaker. Reserve any remaining tincture for another use. Add the ylang-ylang and clary sage essential oils and stir. Pour the mixture through a coffee filter into another glass beaker or container. Using a funnel, pour the filtered liquid into a 1-ounce glass bottle with a fine-mist sprayer. Screw on the top and shake to blend. Label and store in a cool, dark place.

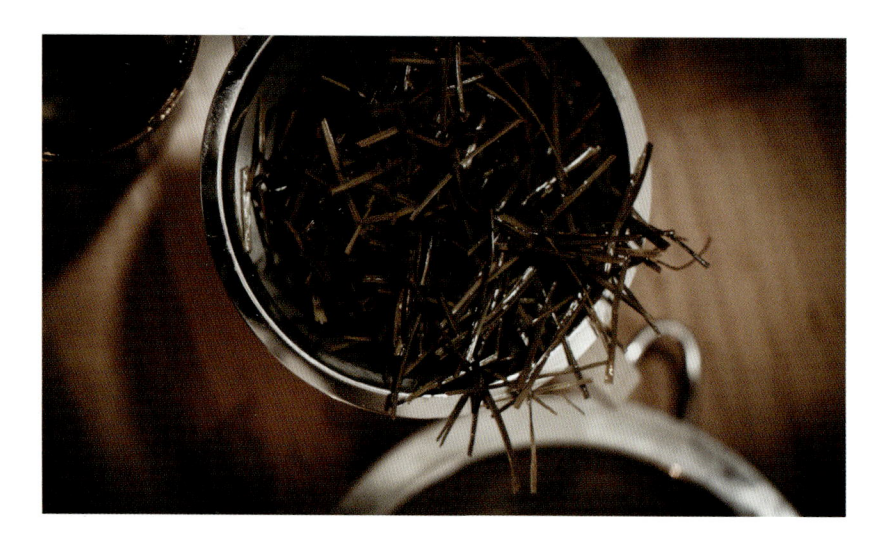

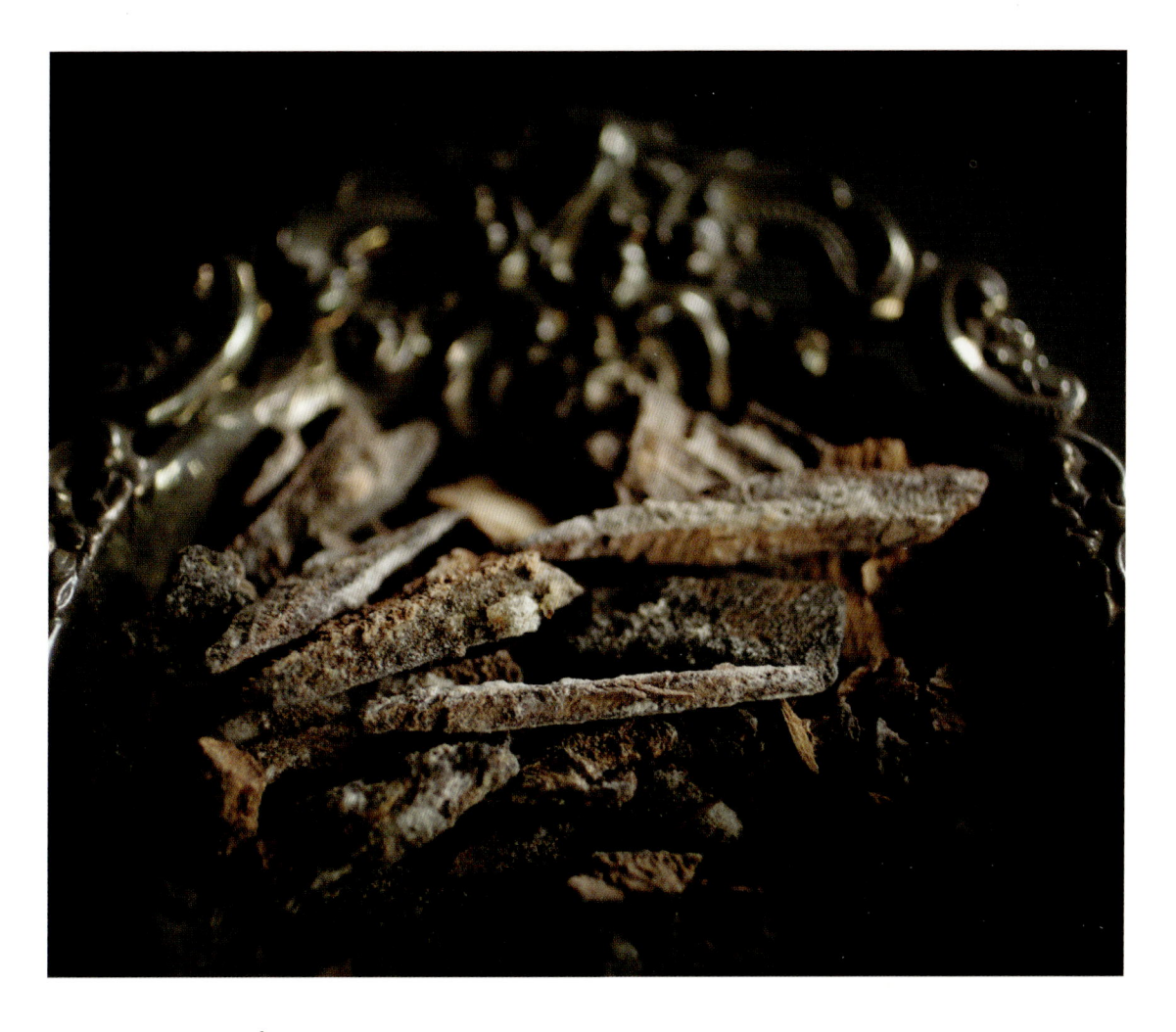

Woods have a quality of strength and stability. If you hug a tree with a wide trunk, you will feel an immediate sense of relief from anxiety. This is because its roots are anchored so far into the earth that it stands absolutely still. It grounds your electrical charge and restores a sense of balance to the nervous system. This is also because wood is a very strong living material and a tree's branches are like protective arms that serve as a perfect shelter for so many creatures. An old tree is the most stable and strong living being—one you may want to befriend.

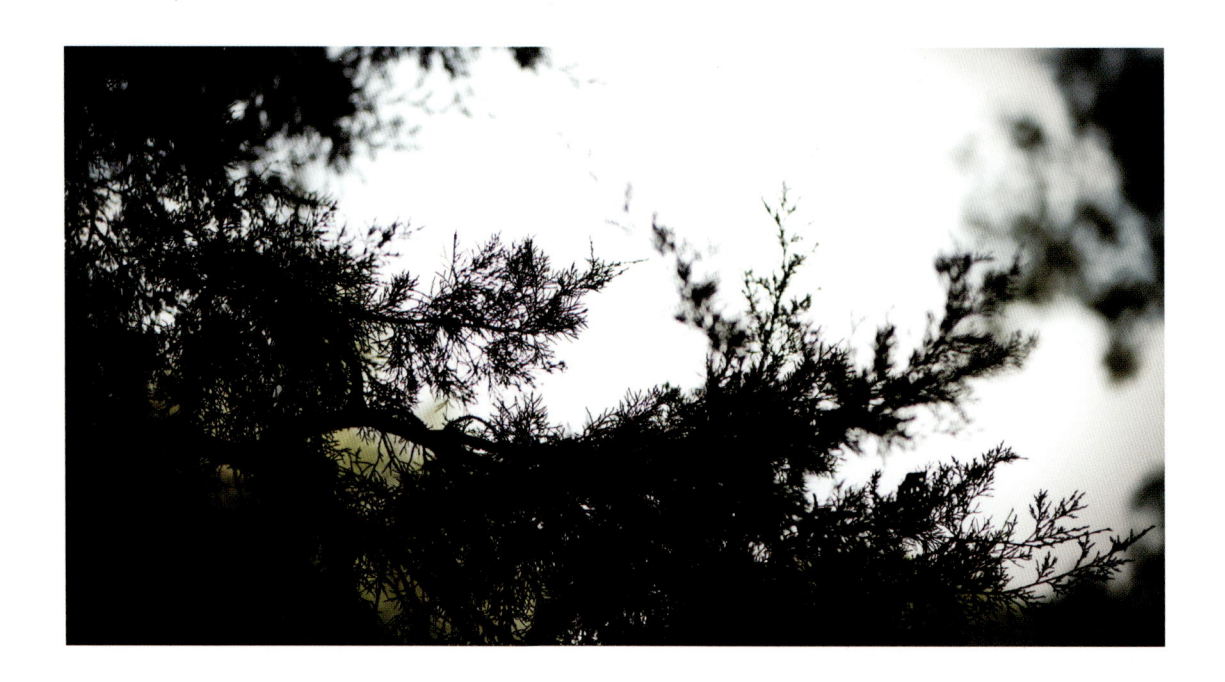

Once, when a sudden hailstorm came over my house, I panicked, realizing that my chickens were outside of their coop. I rushed to the window to discover that they were hiding safely beneath the cedar tree in my yard. After the storm, I thanked the tree and felt lucky to have seen for myself why cedar has such a solid reputation.

CEDAR

Cedar is known across time and cultures for its protective qualities. Its strong scent is itself a protective mechanism against invading insects. Its leaves do not drop; they stay rigid and extended year-round, creating a reliable shelter. In making perfume, I've noticed that many people who gravitate toward cedar as a personal scent are looking to connect with their masculine energy—particularly, the traditionally masculine roles of protector and provider. Cedar essential oil can be irritating to the skin, so it should be diluted to 5 percent or less in a carrier oil or alcohol base. I like it best as incense or room spray to create an aura of protection in my home. True cedars such as the sweet *Cedrus atlantica* and spicy *Cedrus deodara* are often used in perfume; however, the most common and familiar oil is from *Juniperus virginiana*, a juniper known as Eastern red cedar.

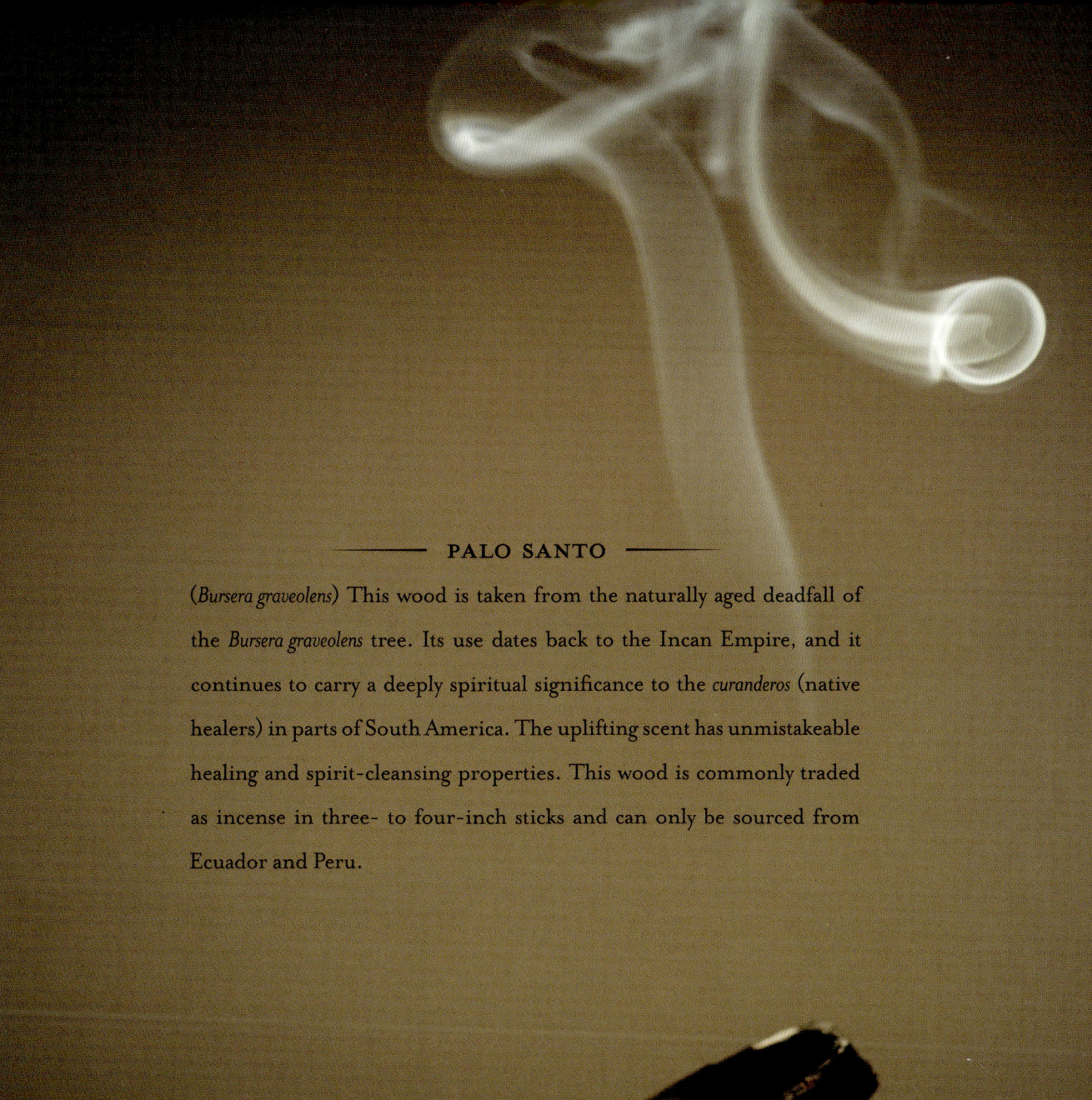

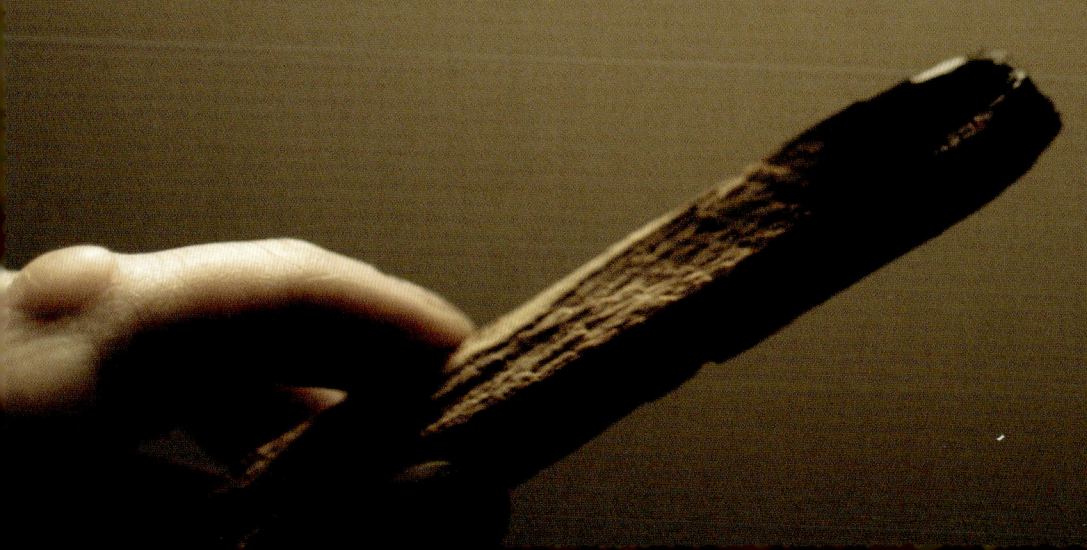

PALO SANTO

(*Bursera graveolens*) This wood is taken from the naturally aged deadfall of the *Bursera graveolens* tree. Its use dates back to the Incan Empire, and it continues to carry a deeply spiritual significance to the *curanderos* (native healers) in parts of South America. The uplifting scent has unmistakeable healing and spirit-cleansing properties. This wood is commonly traded as incense in three- to four-inch sticks and can only be sourced from Ecuador and Peru.

A Note on Sustainability

It is important to source any botanical carefully, as illegal poaching and unsustainable harvesting practices are widespread. Tree products are especially important to source from reliable, ethical harvesters, since trees cannot be replaced quickly. Many wood products for perfume and incense are plantation grown, and ensuring this is essential for products such as sandalwood and agarwood (oud). In the case of palo santo, be sure that it has been properly harvested from aged deadfall. The *Bursera graveolens* lives about sixty years, and its scent does not develop fully in the wood until it has been dead for several years.

Larger threats to trees include climate change issues and agricultural expansion. Often, essential oil producers are invested in the future of their products, and the ethical companies become stewards of the trees, ensuring their land remains forested and protected through sustainable practices.

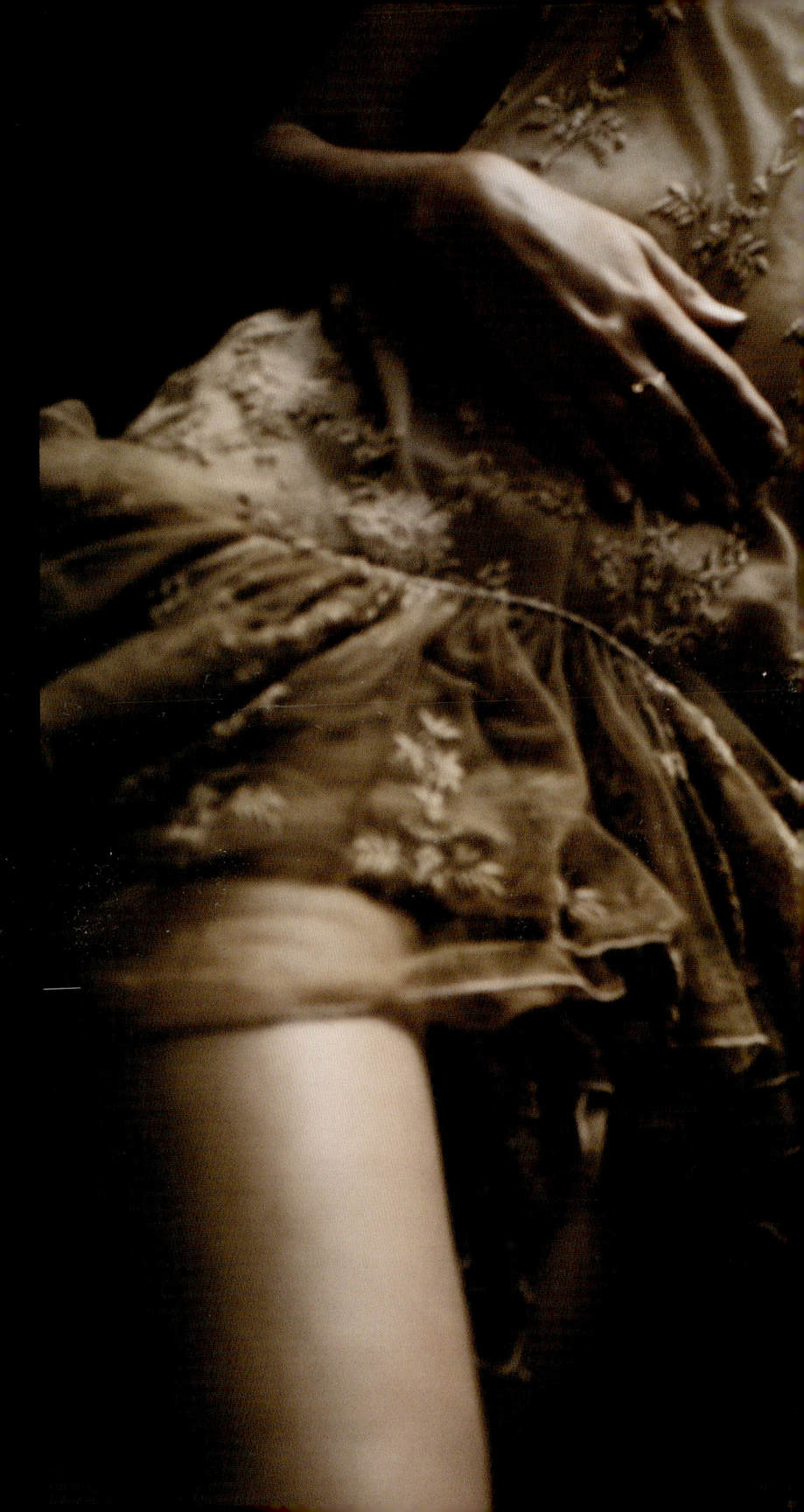

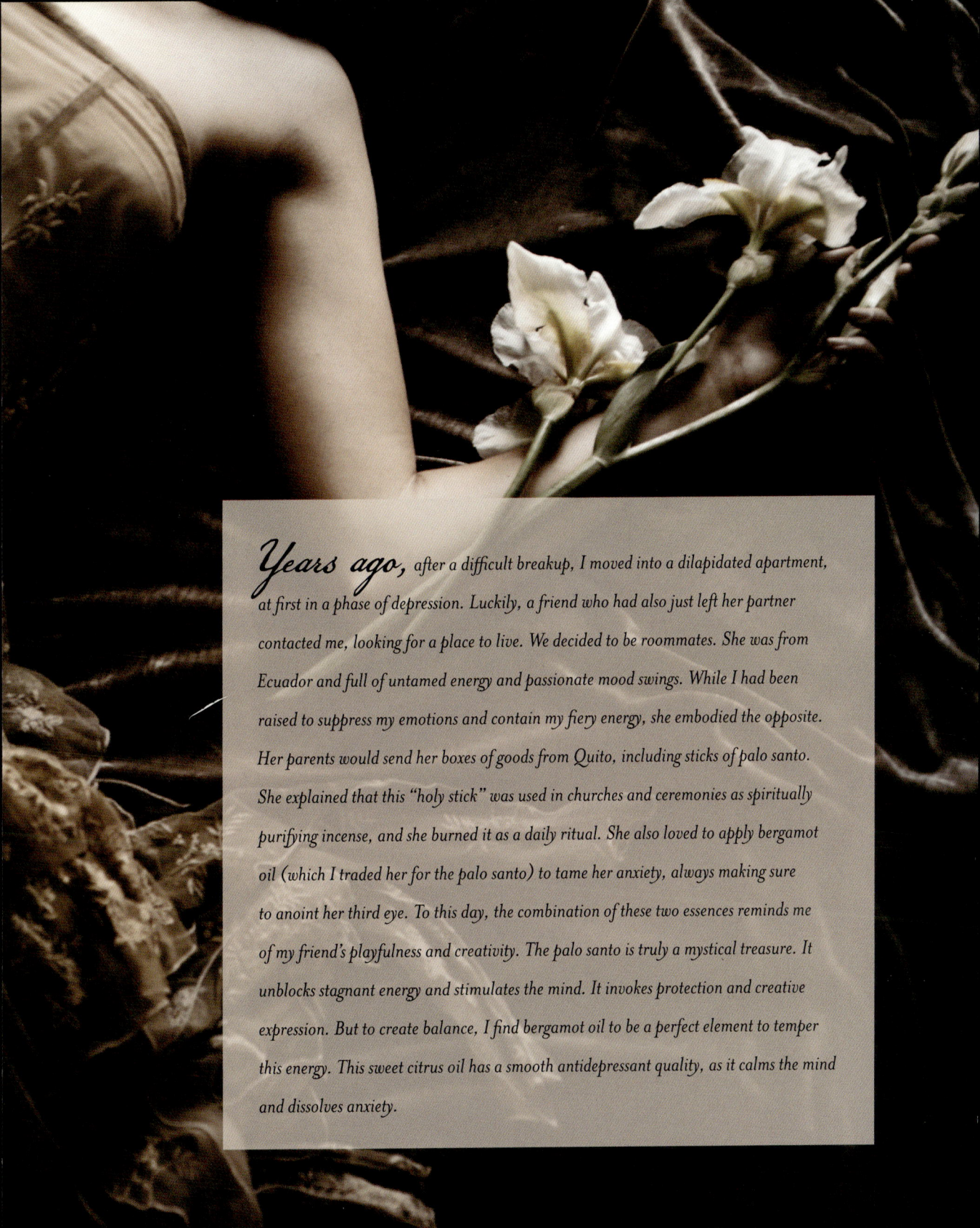

Years ago, after a difficult breakup, I moved into a dilapidated apartment, at first in a phase of depression. Luckily, a friend who had also just left her partner contacted me, looking for a place to live. We decided to be roommates. She was from Ecuador and full of untamed energy and passionate mood swings. While I had been raised to suppress my emotions and contain my fiery energy, she embodied the opposite. Her parents would send her boxes of goods from Quito, including sticks of palo santo. She explained that this "holy stick" was used in churches and ceremonies as spiritually purifying incense, and she burned it as a daily ritual. She also loved to apply bergamot oil (which I traded her for the palo santo) to tame her anxiety, always making sure to anoint her third eye. To this day, the combination of these two essences reminds me of my friend's playfulness and creativity. The palo santo is truly a mystical treasure. It unblocks stagnant energy and stimulates the mind. It invokes protection and creative expression. But to create balance, I find bergamot oil to be a perfect element to temper this energy. This sweet citrus oil has a smooth antidepressant quality, as it calms the mind and dissolves anxiety.

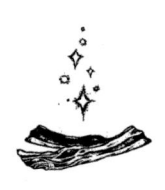

PALO SANTO ENERGY-UNBLOCKING PERFUME

Makes 1 ounce

PALO SANTO TINCTURE

4 to 8 (4-inch) palo santo sticks (or ¼ cup chipped pieces)

190-proof organic alcohol

PERFUME

25 milliliters palo santo tincture

20 drops bergamot essential oil*

10 drops frankincense essential oil

5 milliliters orange blossom water (hydrosol) or plain distilled water

*Bergamot oil is photosensitizing and should be diluted with a carrier oil to less than 5 percent before being applied to the skin. To anoint the third eye, use a special bergamot oil that has the bergapten molecule removed. This reduces its phototoxicity and only slightly alters its scent.

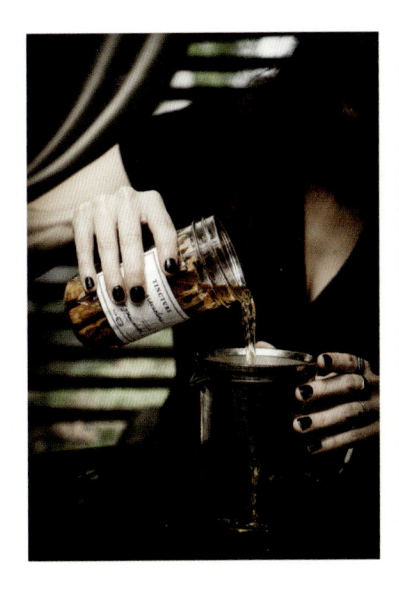

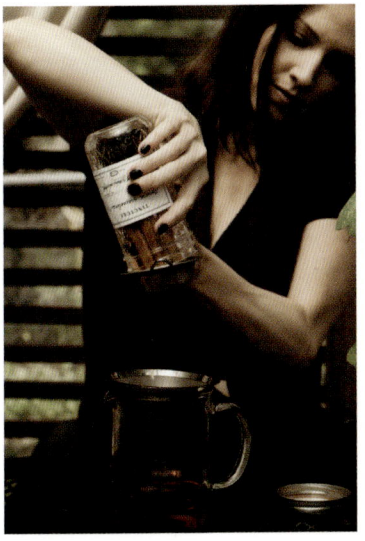

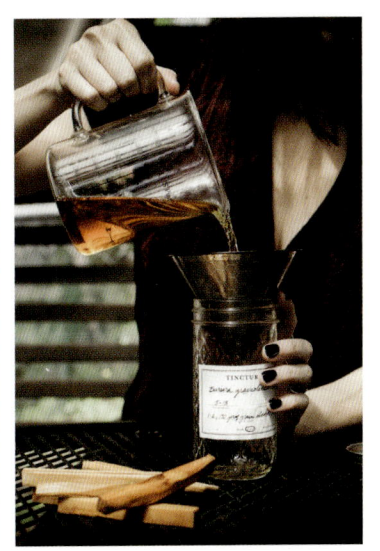

To make the palo santo tincture, place the palo santo sticks in an 8 to 12-ounce glass jar with an airtight lid. Pour in enough alcohol to cover the wood completely. Seal and allow to tincture for 3 weeks, shaking occasionally. Pour the tincture through a fine-mesh strainer or cheesecloth. (Reserve the palo santo sticks, as they will still be fragrant; once the alcohol has evaporated from them, they can be burned as incense.) Seal the tincture in the jar. Label it and store in a cool, dark place.

To make the perfume, combine 25 milliliters of the palo santo tincture (reserving any extra for another use) with the bergamot and frankincense essential oils and the orange blossom water in a 1-ounce glass bottle with a fine-mist sprayer. Screw on the top and shake to blend. Label and store in a cool, dark place.

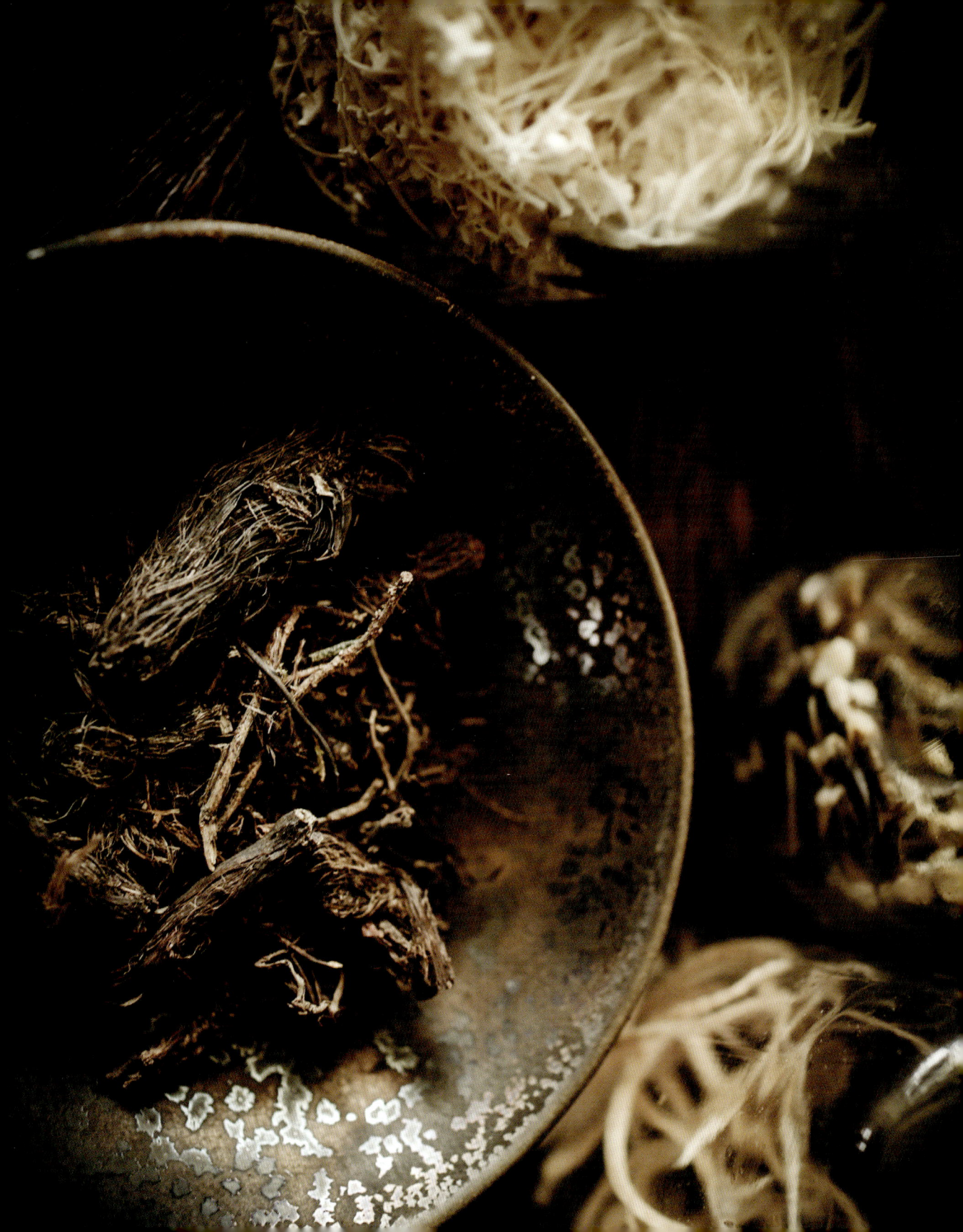

Roots are powerful sources of comfort during times of grief and loss. Grief, a complex emotional state, feels to me as if my roots have been ripped out from beneath me and my body is floating above ground, vulnerable to the slightest wind. I forget how to take in nourishment, and I'm severed from my normal routines.

I have noticed that the deep, dark nature of root essential oils offers a sense of resolution when no true closure exists. Their scents are bold and earthy, requiring you to spend some time to acclimate to them. As you become familiar with a root, you may notice yourself feeling a strong sense of relief and reconnection to your own sense of ground. Some roots, such as ginger, settle the stomach when it feels uneasy; others, like valerian, have a sedative effect, soothing the unsettled parts of our subconscious. Angelica root is used as a women's tonic in traditional Chinese medicine, an uplifting and emotionally supportive charm in American folk magic, and was associated with the protective archangel Michael in medieval Europe. I like to blend it with other selected root oils to create custom aromatic talismans.

A Note on Sustainability

Harvesting roots and rhizomes can be destructive to the plant, and wild-harvesting roots is usually not sustainable. Organically cultivated roots are a more sustainable option, and I encourage using the oils conservatively. This means candles, soaps, and other products that use large amounts of essential oil are not appropriate for root oils. (This is true of many other essential oils as well.) Luckily, roots have such a strong scent that a couple drops can last months in an aromatherapy inhaler. They also have a long shelf life and can be worn sparingly as perfume.

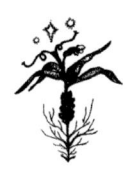

HEALING ROOTS AROMATHERAPY INHALER

2 drops angelica root essential oil

1 drop vetiver essential oil

Fill a lip balm tube with a cotton ball or other absorbent natural fiber. Add the angelica and vetiver essential oils to the cotton. This inhaler will last up to a year if stored in a cool, dark place.

To use throughout the day as needed, or during meditation, remove the lid and hold the tube below your nose; inhale deeply.

VETIVER

(*Vetiveria zizanoides*) This grass originates in India and is grown in several regions with hot climates. Its roots, which grow as deep as 13 feet into the ground, contain more than 150 aromatic compounds. Vetiver root is soothing and sweet, comforting and relaxing. It tempers anger and heat. It allows us to open to our vulnerabilities, extend our patience, and feel a deep-rooted support that facilitates healing.

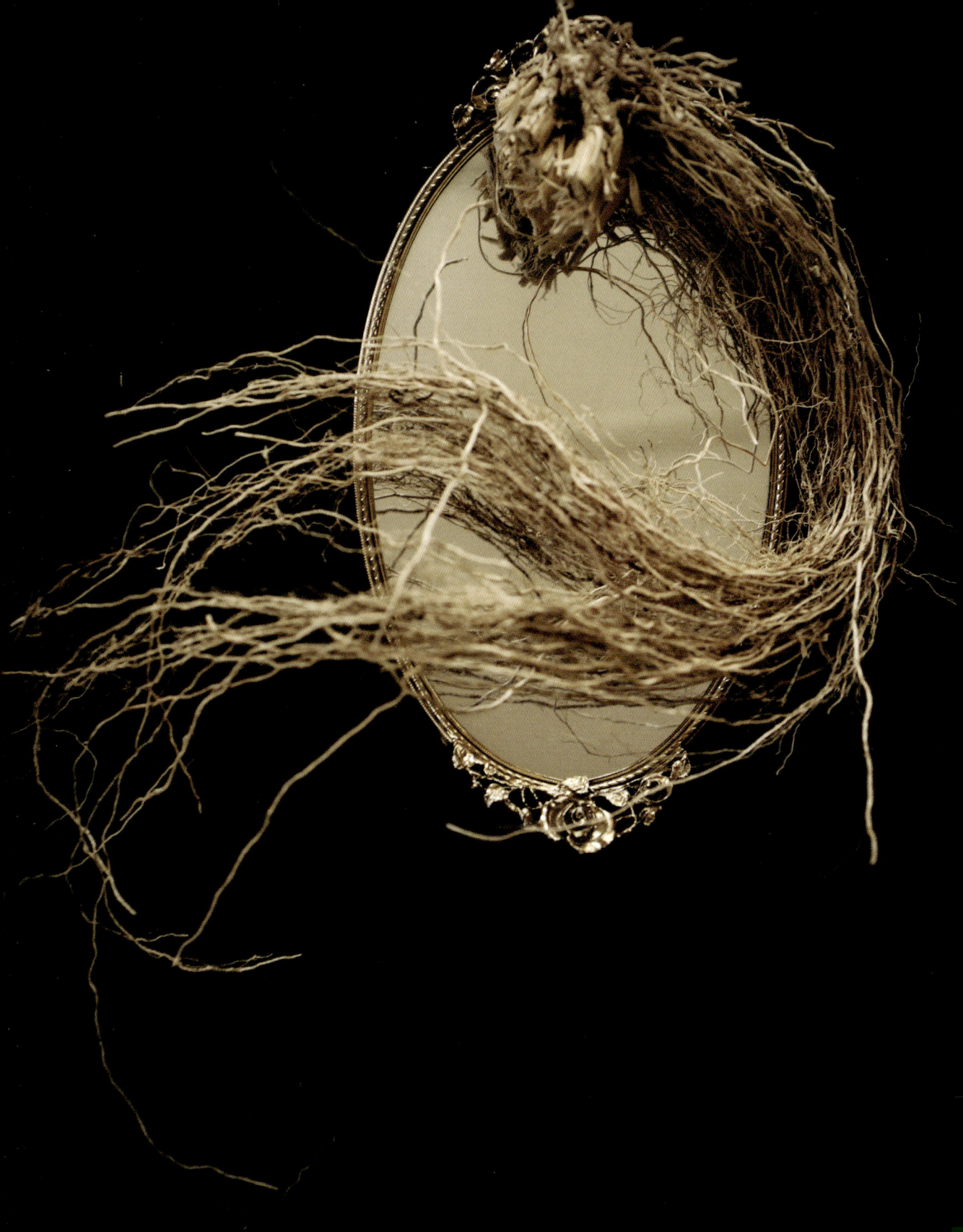

VETIVER HEALING SALVE

Makes about 2 ounces

NOTE: For this recipe, you will need a 2-ounce jar with an airtight lid or several smaller containers.

½ ounce (by weight) frankincense resin, frozen*

1 fluid ounce jojoba oil*

½ ounce (by weight) beeswax, grated

30 drops vetiver essential oil

*Freezing the resin before grinding it makes it less sticky.

*Since jojoba oil is actually a liquid wax, not an oil, it will not turn rancid, so this salve won't expire.

Using a mortar and pestle, crush the frankincense resin.

Pour the jojoba oil into a double boiler and add the crushed frankincense resin; heat to about 200°F. Stir occasionally, allowing the frankincense to infuse in the jojoba oil for 30 minutes. (Alternatively, microwave the jojoba oil to about 200°F in a glass liquid measuring cup or beaker, then stir in the frankincense resin, allowing it to infuse while cooling for 30 minutes.)

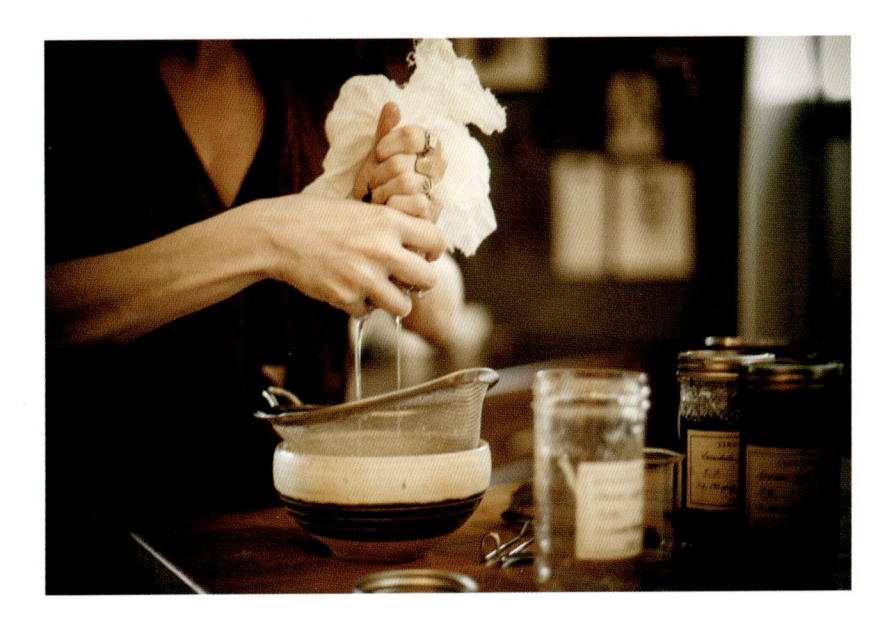

Pour the oil through a fine-mesh strainer or cheesecloth and discard the remaining frankincense gum (or reserve to burn as incense). Add the beeswax to the mixture and return to the heat until the wax melts.

Remove from the heat, allowing to cool (but not solidify) for about 2 minutes. Add the vetiver essential oil and stir. Using a funnel, pour into a 2-ounce glass jar with an airtight lid or several smaller containers. Label and store sealed in a cool, dark place.

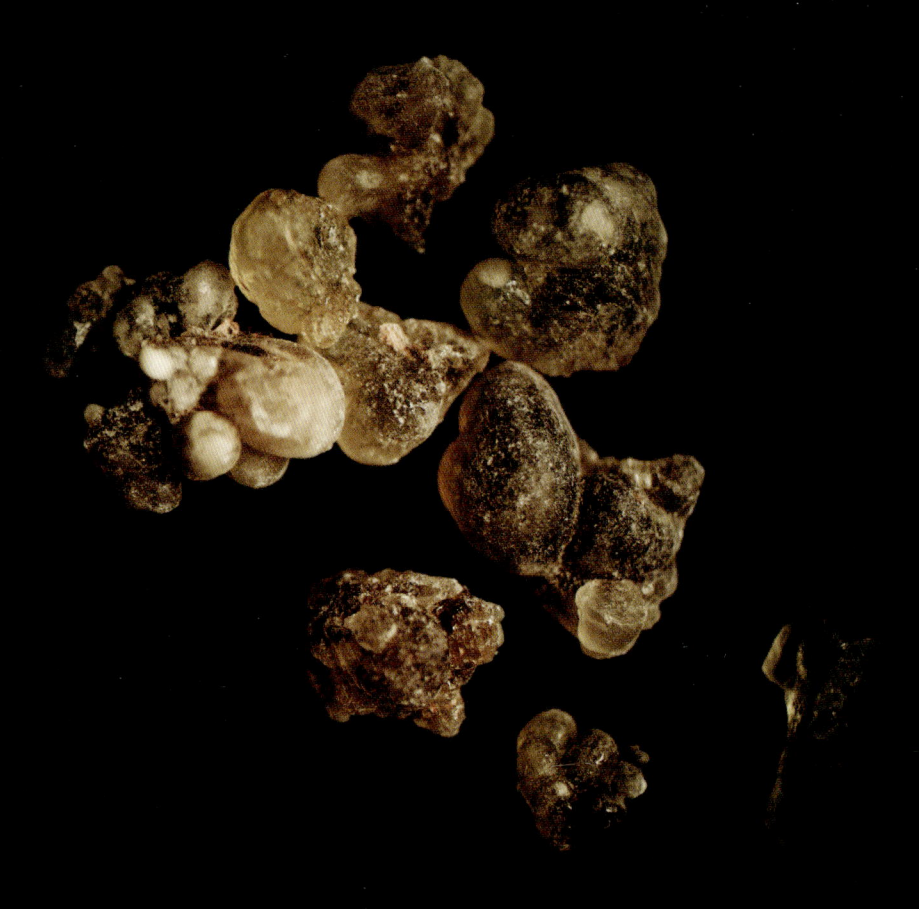

Resins heal the wounds of trees, and they can do the same for us. The antimicrobial materials in resins can protect skin abrasions, and similarly, the sweet, comforting scent of the essential oils they contain has a healing effect on emotional wounds. I like to use a hint of resin in my incense blends because its sweet, honey-like quality allows the darker wood and spice elements to open up. We need some sweetness in order to fully appreciate the dark notes. Many resins burn beautifully as incense on charcoal if they are crushed into small pieces first. My favorites for burning on charcoal are hojari frankincense, white copal, and myrrh.

Tree Resin Tips

- A convenient way to use tree resins as incense is to place a piece of foil on an electric mug warmer (a mini warming plate) and then place the resin on top of the foil. The heat of the warmer plate will not create smoke, but it will still distribute the scent. This method does not require as much careful attention and still has many of the aromatic benefits.

- When adding tree resins to your loose incense blends, remember that they are very sticky. To make crushing easier, put the resin in a container and place it in the freezer for a few hours. Then use a mortar and pestle to grind the frozen resin. Tree exudates are oleo-gum-resins, which means they not only contain resins but also oil-soluble gum, and both the gum and resin contain essential oils. The resin is the hard, clearer part.

- Tree resins are likely to stick to the pan while simmering and to your other tools when you are working with them. The gum is soluble in oil, and the resin can be cleaned easily with alcohol.

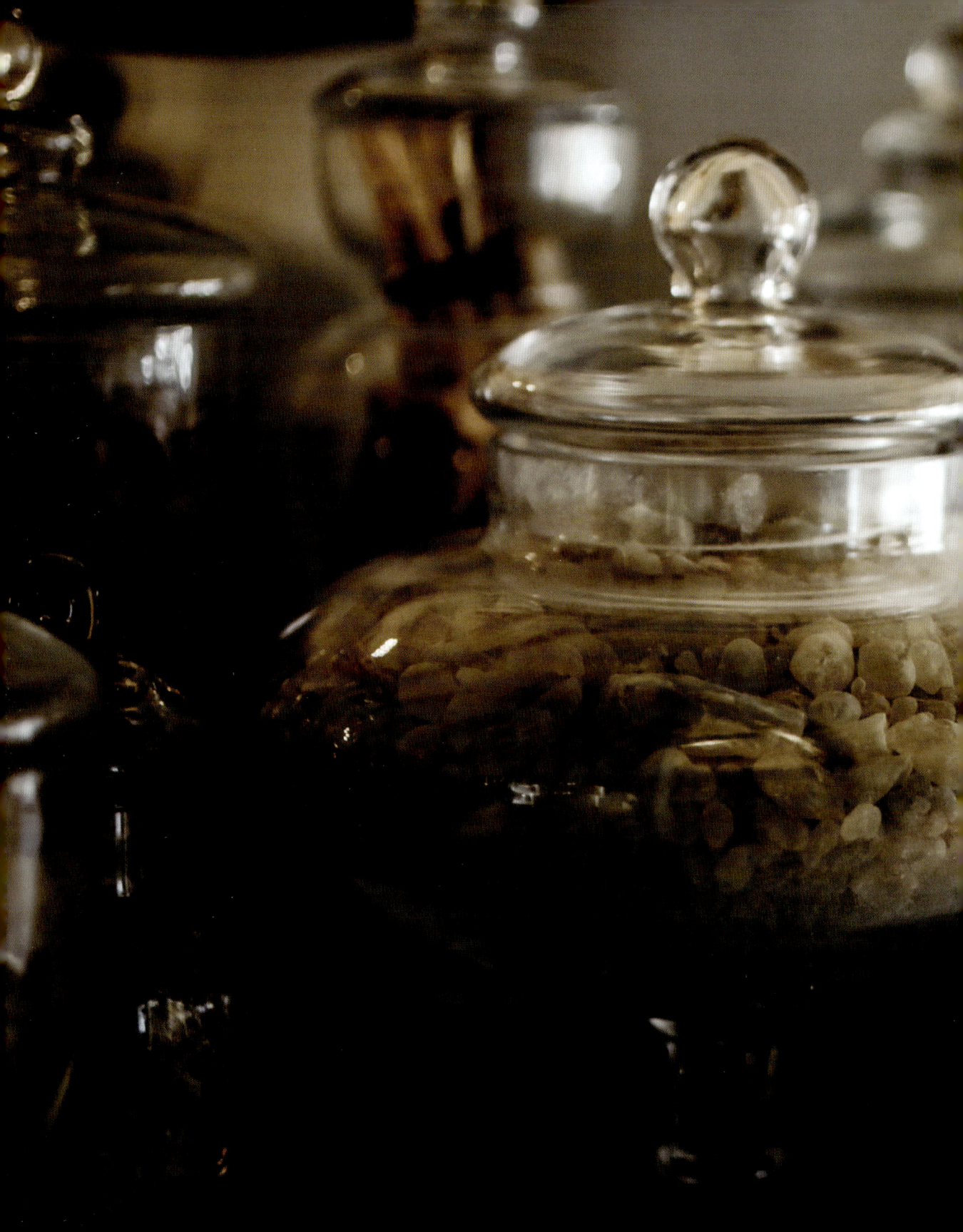

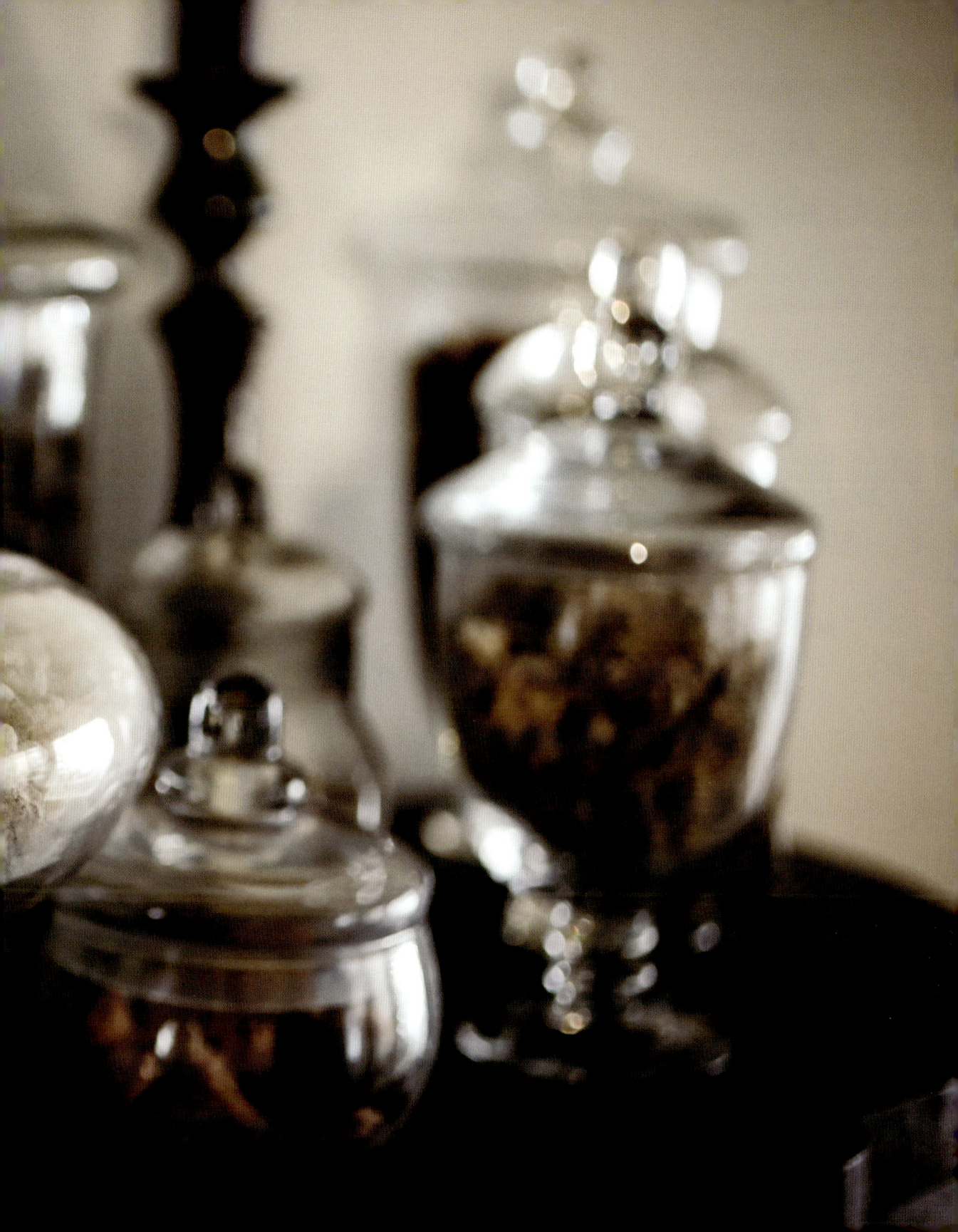

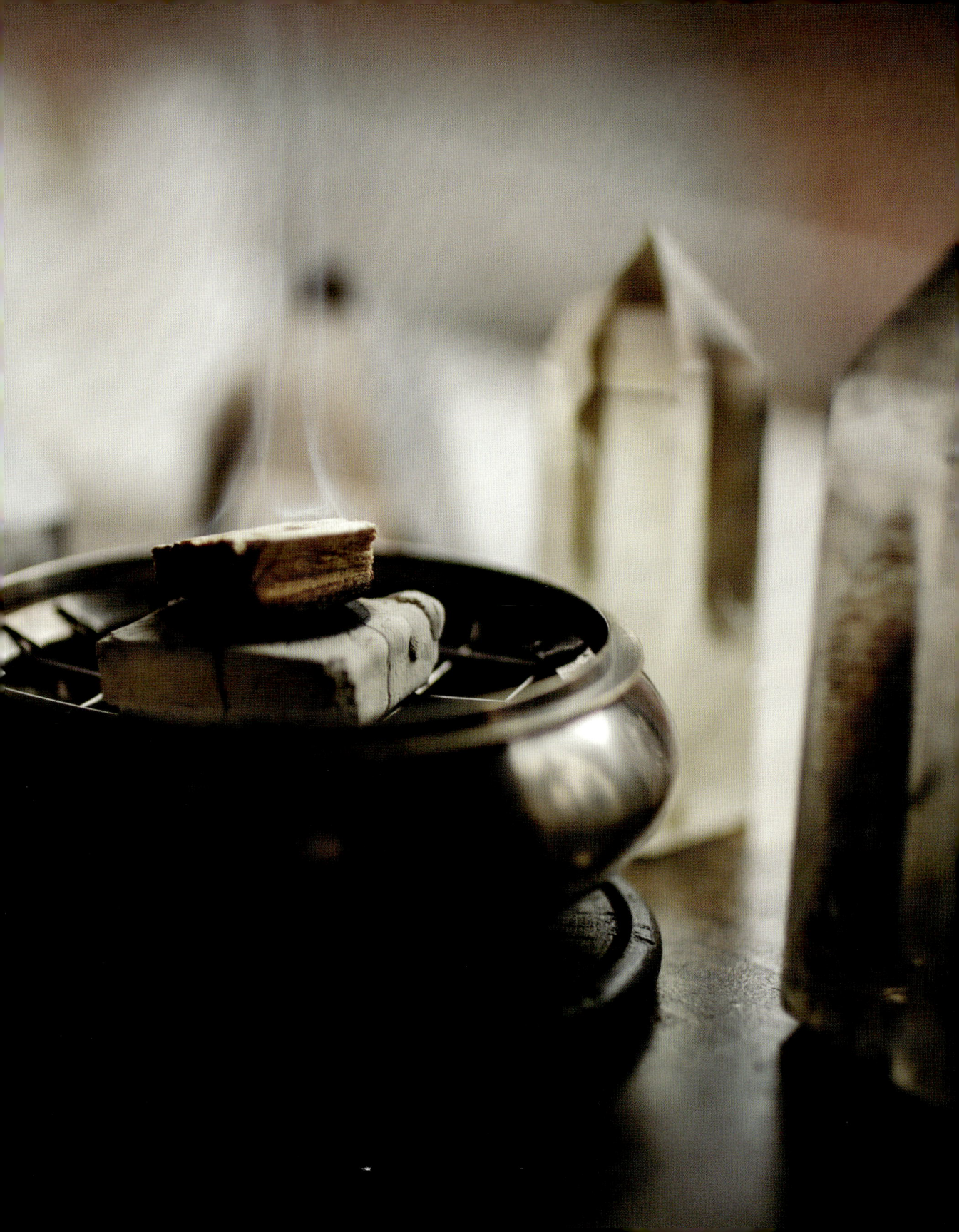

Six

INCENSE

Incense is the foundation of natural perfume, as the word "perfume" comes from the Latin words *per*, meaning "through," and *fume*, meaning "smoke." For thousands of years, in cultures around the globe, aromatic woods, resins, and other plant materials have been burned ceremonially, often as offerings to the gods and ancestors. When these precious materials are burned, the aromatic smoke they create becomes a part of the spirit world, creating a bridge between the realms.

Any environment, and the energy of those within it, can be transformed by infusing the air with an aromatic plant. Intentionally filling a space with smoke, leaving behind invisible scent, is understood in virtually every culture to be a spiritually cleansing practice. But not all incense is equal, and when we work with incense, we are not simply smelling the scented air it creates; we are consuming the plant itself through our lungs and limbic system. Much like synthetic perfume, synthetic incense includes chemical binders, burning agents, and fragrances that can be toxic to ingest. Although there are some beautiful and clean natural incense sticks, cones, and coils available, I like to make my own loose incense blends from natural materials at home. Making homemade incense allows me to connect more deeply with the materials through hand-blending them. It also frees me to create blends that are meaningful to me based on the careful acquisition of the materials and the significance each ingredient holds for me spiritually.

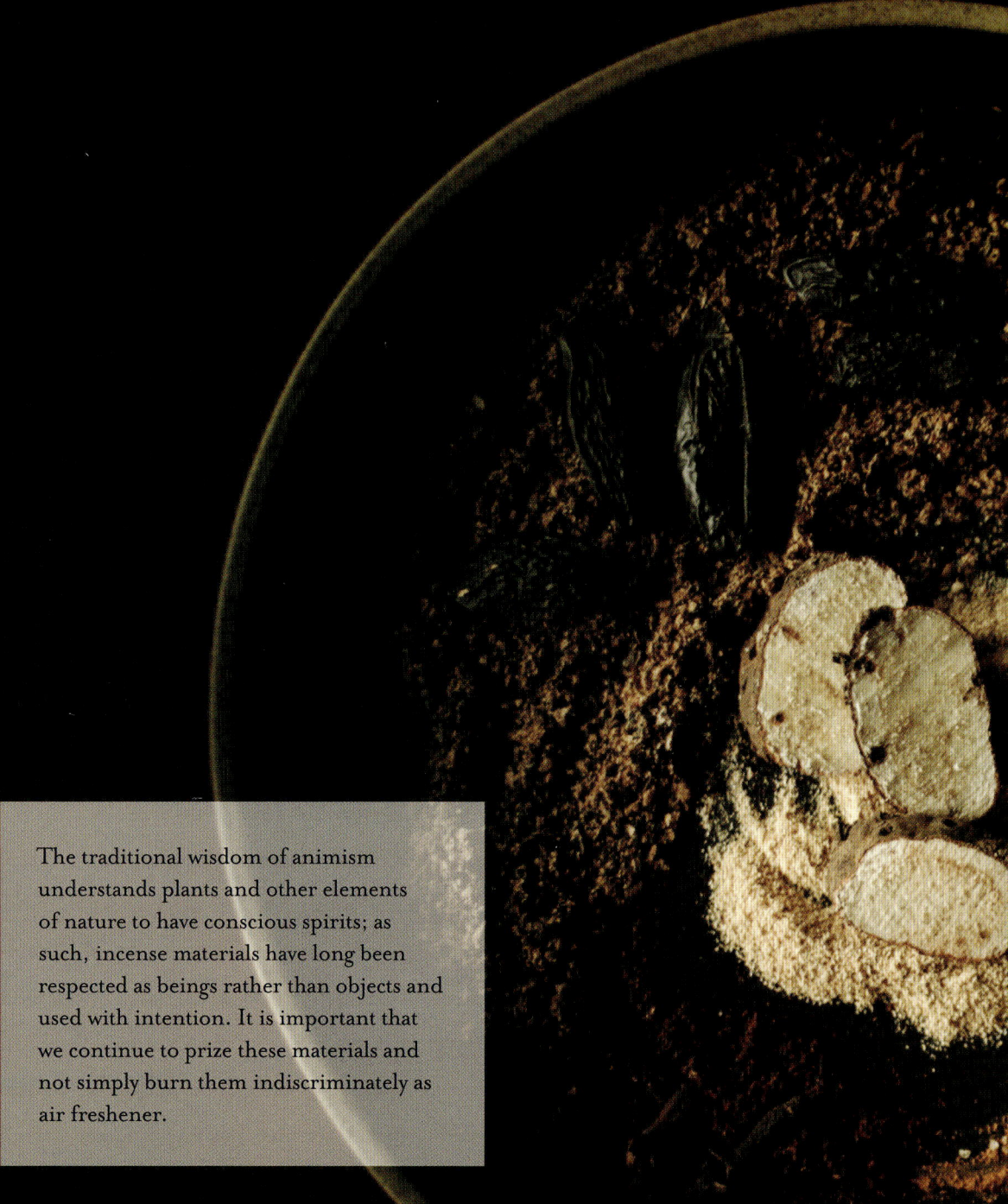

The traditional wisdom of animism understands plants and other elements of nature to have conscious spirits; as such, incense materials have long been respected as beings rather than objects and used with intention. It is important that we continue to prize these materials and not simply burn them indiscriminately as air freshener.

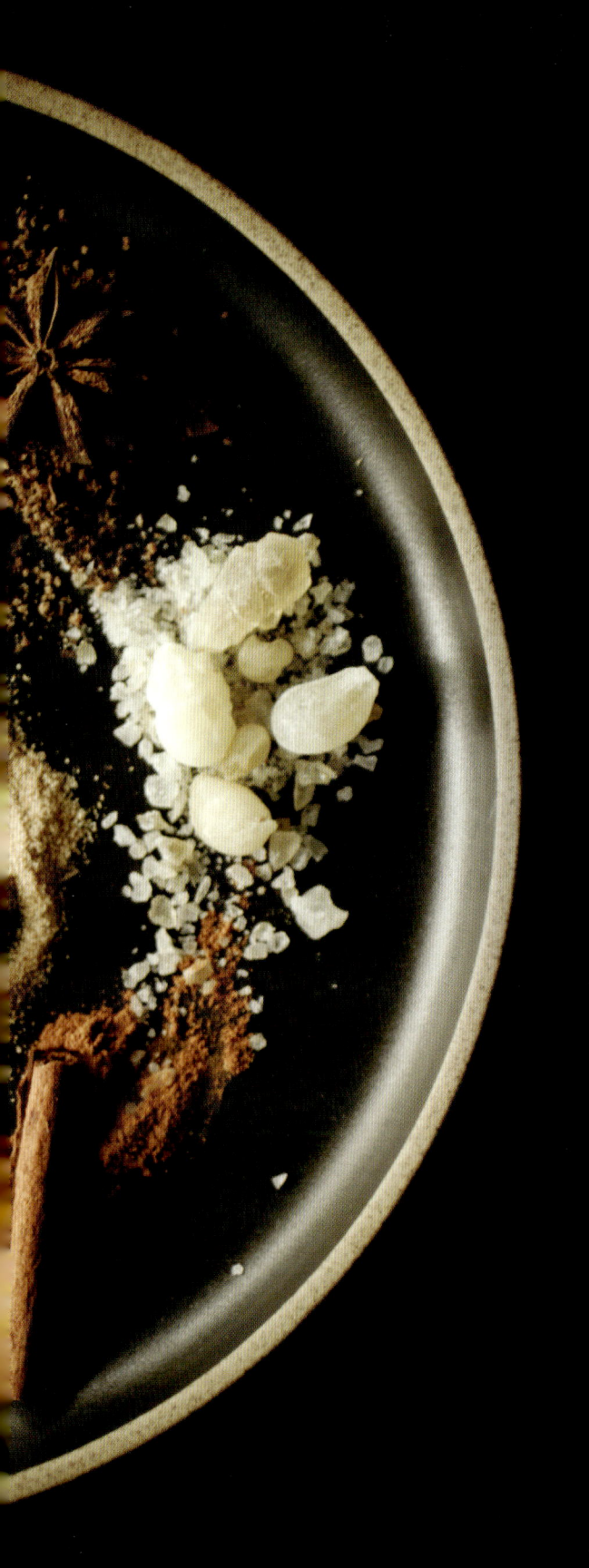

How to Burn Loose Incense

Loose incense is most commonly burned over charcoal. I like to use bamboo charcoal from Japan, as this is the cleanest-burning kind I have found. Many other charcoals contain saltpeter and other chemicals that degrade the purity and scent of the natural incense.

Heat the charcoal over a flame and place in a small bowl of ash or sand, or as I prefer, on the screen of a *bakhoor* burner. The edges of the charcoal will begin to turn white as the heat distributes. If you are burning delicate materials, you might want to add a thin layer of salt over the surface of the charcoal to reduce the heat, then place a small spoonful of loose incense on top. Make sure your incense material is coarsely ground and relatively uniform in size, as larger pieces will not burn evenly.

Once the smoke has settled and the material has burned, use tongs to brush the used botanicals off the charcoal and place a new layer of incense on the cleaned charcoal.

I first encountered Artemisia tridentata *during a trip to northern New Mexico. I returned for a summer, years later, to build sustainable architecture with Earthship Biotecture. From the balcony of the Earthship I lived in north of Taos, I could see big sagebrush stretching to the horizon. When the rain came over the mesa, the essential oils of this high desert native were released into the air, filling the atmosphere with the scent of peace and purification. Thanks in part to the presence of this herb, my summer in New Mexico was therapeutic during a time when I had been haunted; I was off the grid, surrounded and supported by the sagebrush's spirit.*

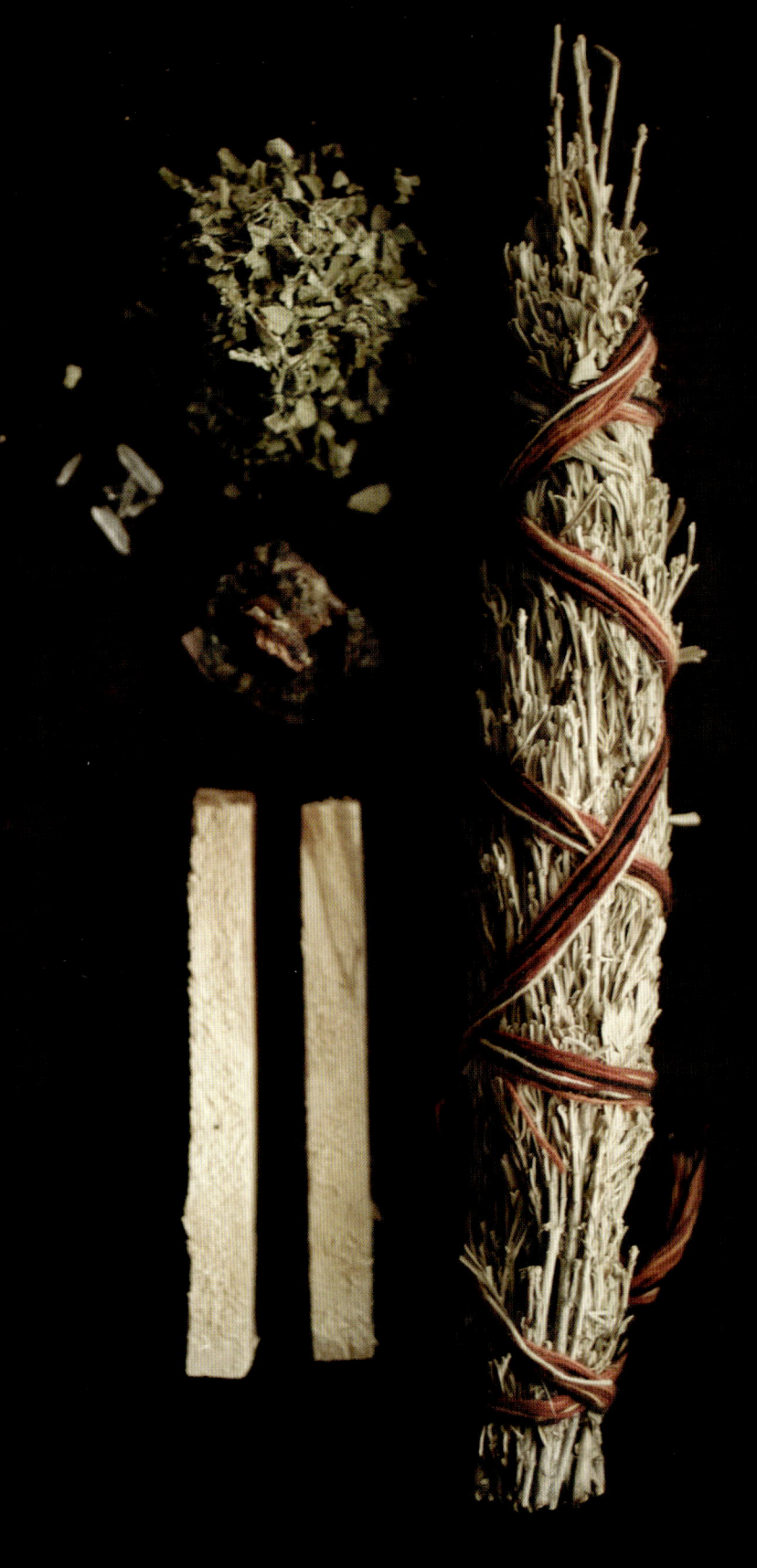

I like to burn the following five botanicals over charcoal or as dried wands in new home, new moon, and new beginning rituals. Any combination of these is excellent for psychic protection as well as recalibrating the energy of a space.

PALO SANTO

(Bursera graveolens) As I've already mentioned, I adore this aromatic wood. Its essence carries high energy, spirit healing and cleansing properties, and it unlocks the creative mind. Palo santo is commonly sold as incense in three- to four-inch-long sticks.

BIG SAGEBRUSH

(Artemisia tridentata) This fragrant herb has long been used in smudge wands by Native Americans to drive out malevolent spirits and influences, and its purifying scent creates a powerful energy of renewal. It smells like a dark, dry sage with hints of camphor and a smooth, spicy undertone. I find its scent to be tenacious and soothing.

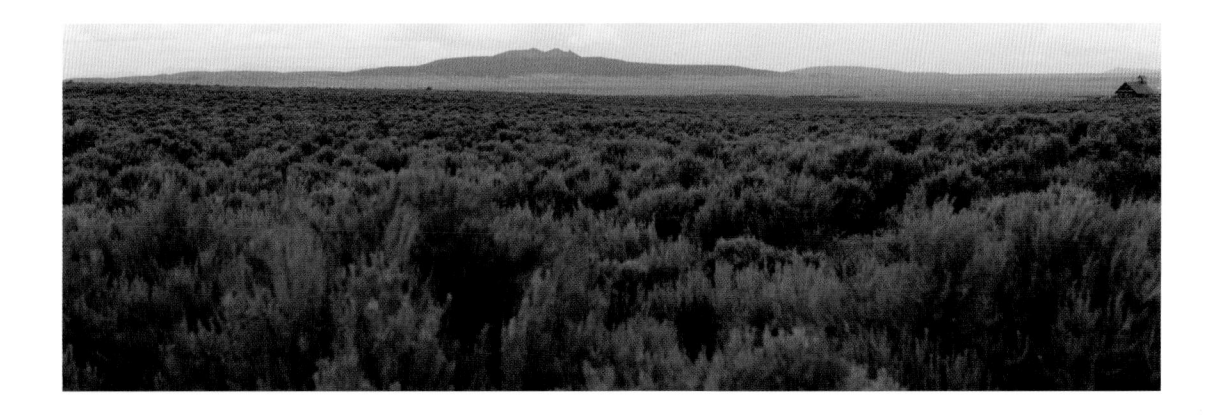

SWEETGRASS

(*Hierochloe odorata*) The comforting scent of sweetgrass (whose botanical name translates to "fragrant holy grass") invites good spirits with a soft essence reminiscent of warm vanilla and alfalfa. Native to both Europe and North America, it grows in cool meadows and near water sources, and it has been recognized as sacred in many cultures. Traditionally, sweetgrass was placed on the floors of Northern European churches on saints' days, and Native Americans continue to use it to make baskets, amulets, and, of course, a peace-inducing incense.

YERBA SANTA

(*Eriodictyon angustifolium*) Yerba santa is an evergreen native to the southwestern United States, dubbed "holy weed" by Spanish priests when they were introduced to the herb's many medicinal properties by Native Californians. Burning it as incense is believed to help protect our emotional boundaries and strengthen the heart energetically. Its scent is deep green, bitter, and resinous, with a medicinal undertone.

EASTERN RED CEDAR

(*Juniperus virginiana*) There are many varieties of cedar, but Eastern red cedar, which is technically a juniper but respected as a cedar, is my favorite to use. This essential oil is easy to find because it's produced from the leftover wood scraps from the pencil and lumber industries. The strength of this rich wood is revealed in its aroma, which offers a powerful sense of protection.

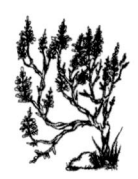

INCENSE BLEND FOR SPIRIT CLEANSING, PROTECTION, AND STRENGTH

Makes about ⅓ cup of loose incense (or 36 uses)

1 stick or ¼ ounce precut palo santo chips

2 tablespoons big sagebrush, dried, cut into ½-inch pieces

1 tablespoon yerba santa, dried, crushed

5 drops Virginia cedar essential oil

1 tablespoon sweetgrass, dried, cut into ½-inch pieces

Small pinch menthol crystals, crushed (optional)

Using a small saw, cut the palo santo stick into ½-inch pieces (if using precut chips, skip this step).

Place all ingredients in a 4-ounce glass jar with an airtight lid and seal. Shake, allowing the elements to blend together and the oil to absorb.

Burn half a teaspoon of this mixture on bamboo charcoal as incense (see "How to Burn Loose Incense," page 71).

The previous incense blend, and any of the incense blends in this book, can be tinctured and made into a room–linen–body mist as shown in the next recipe. If being made for that use, note that any resins and resinous leaves such as yerba santa should be omitted, because they will clog the spray nozzles. If finely ground herbs are used in the tincture, it will need to be strained through a coffee filter before bottling.

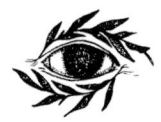

PSYCHIC CLEANSING ROOM–LINEN–BODY MIST

Makes 6 to 8 ounces

This mist is one I love to make and use in my own home.

TINCTURE

3 thin palo santo sticks

¼ cup dried big sagebrush

¼ cup dried sweetgrass

Organic 190-proof alcohol or organic vodka

ROOM–LINEN–BODY MIST

30 drops (about 1 milliliter) Virginia cedarwood essential oil

2 ounces distilled water

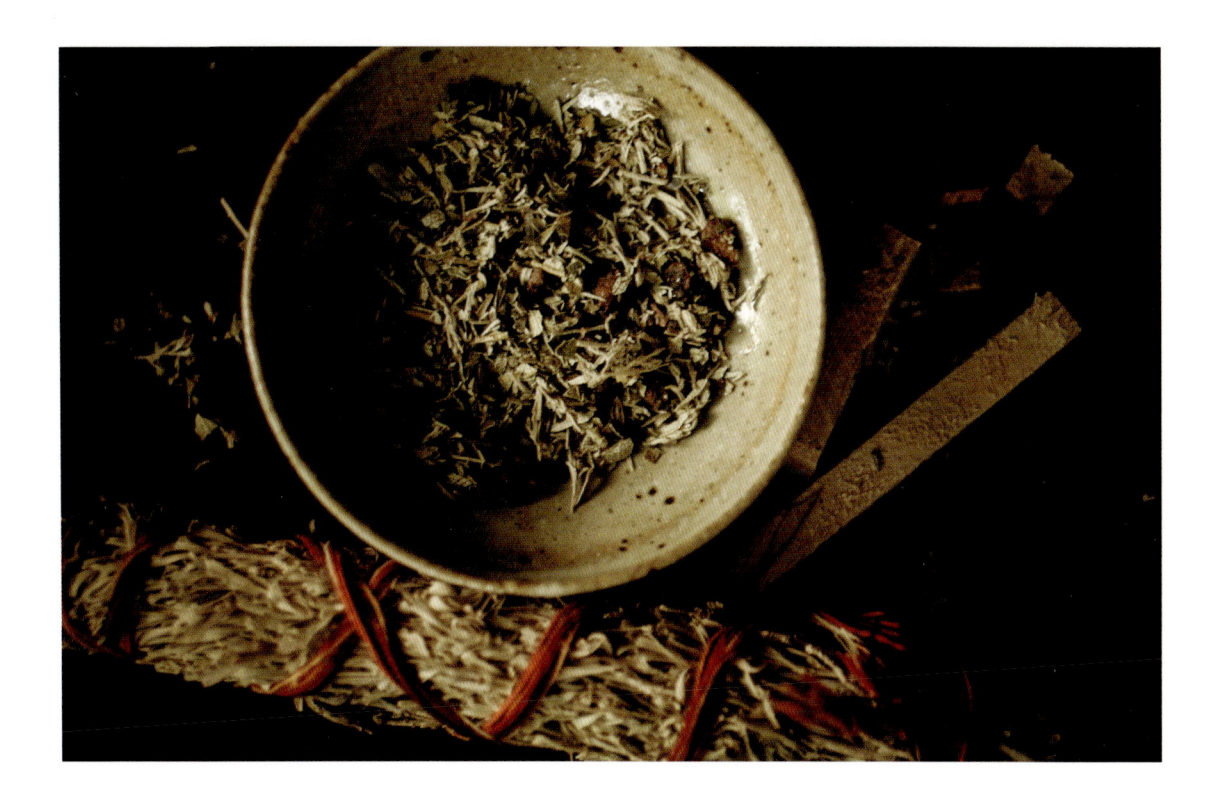

To make the tincture, combine the palo santo sticks, big sagebrush, and sweetgrass in a 12-ounce glass jar with an airtight lid. Pour in enough alcohol to cover the botanicals completely and seal. Allow the mixture to tincture for at least 2 weeks if using 190-proof spirits and at least 4 weeks if using the vodka. Pour the tincture through a fine-mesh strainer or cheesecloth into a clean container, discarding the botanicals. (Reserve the palo santo sticks, which can be burned as incense after drying.)

To make the mist, add the Virginia cedarwood essential oil to the tincture. Add the distilled water if 190-proof alcohol was used in the tincture (skip if vodka was used in the tincture). Using a funnel, pour the mixture into an 8-ounce glass spray bottle or several smaller spray bottles. Screw on the top and shake to blend. Label and store in a cool, dark place.

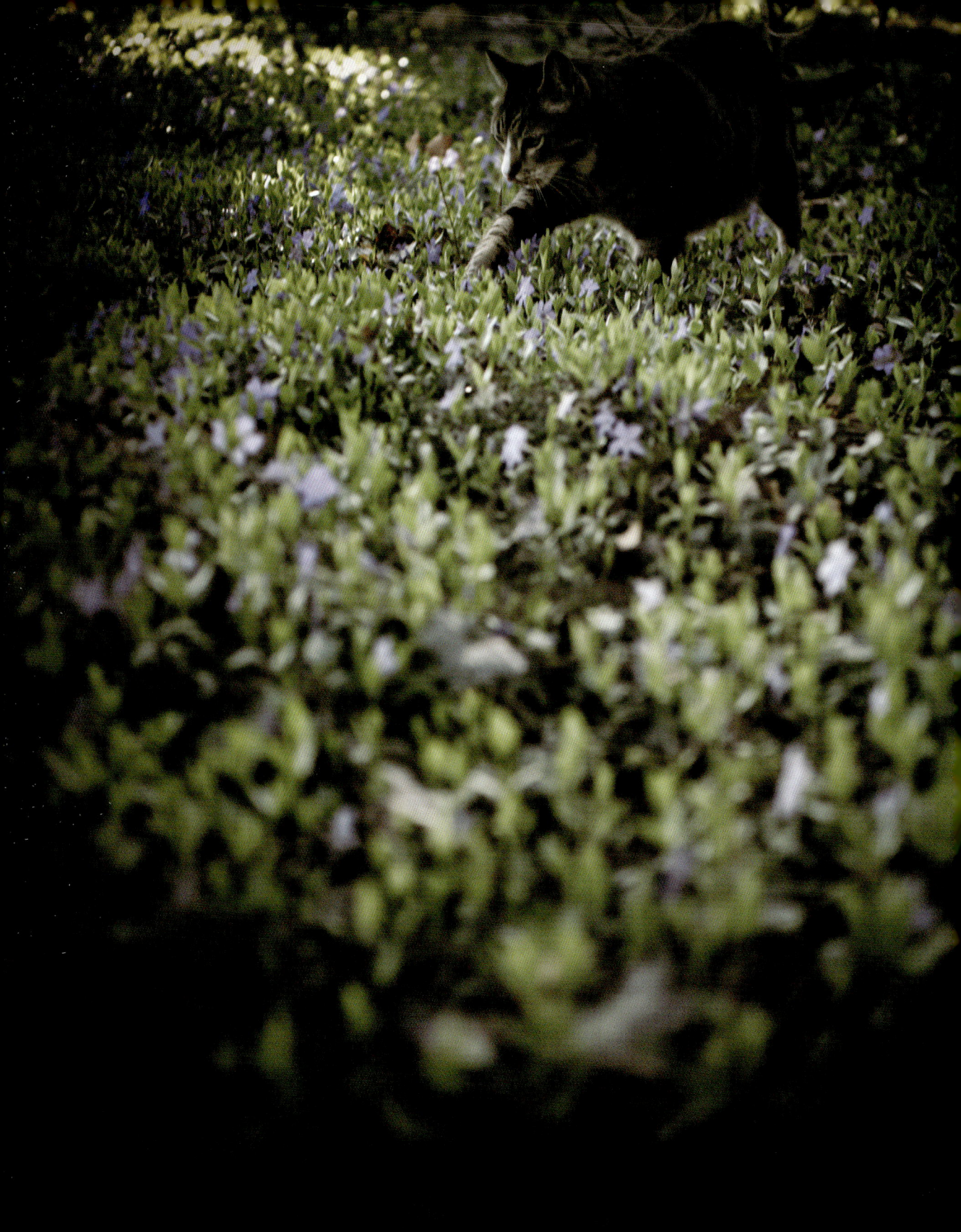

Seven

WELCOMING THE SEASONS

I find that living in a four-season climate is essential to my connection with nature. The seasons themselves comfort me with senses of change and progress, rest and growth, and ritual and routine. I am attuned to which flowers bloom at what times throughout the year, their predictability assuring me that everything is as it should be.

Autumn

Autumn brings the harvest. There's a race to gather the final fruits of the year's labor, and then to dry, preserve, and store them for the winter. (Because most of us no longer homestead, this autumnal hoarding impulse often expresses itself as frenzied holiday shopping.) As the days get cooler and shorter, we naturally crave spicy, warm drinks and larger cooked meals to help us adjust to the environment.

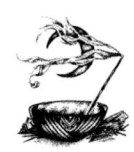

AUTUMN EQUINOX LOOSE INCENSE

Makes about ¼ cup of loose incense (or 24 uses)

I love bringing the warmth and coziness of autumn into my home with candles and incense. This incense blend is my favorite for welcoming the autumn equinox in mid-September.

2 teaspoons clove powder

4 teaspoons ground tonka bean (or vanilla powder)

2 teaspoons ground star anise

2 teaspoons ground frankincense

1 teaspoon cassia powder

1 teaspoon orris root powder

Combine the clove powder, tonka bean, star anise, frankincense, cassia powder, and orris root powder in a small bowl, blending well.

Burn half a teaspoon of this mixture on bamboo charcoal as incense (see "How to Burn Loose Incense," page 71).

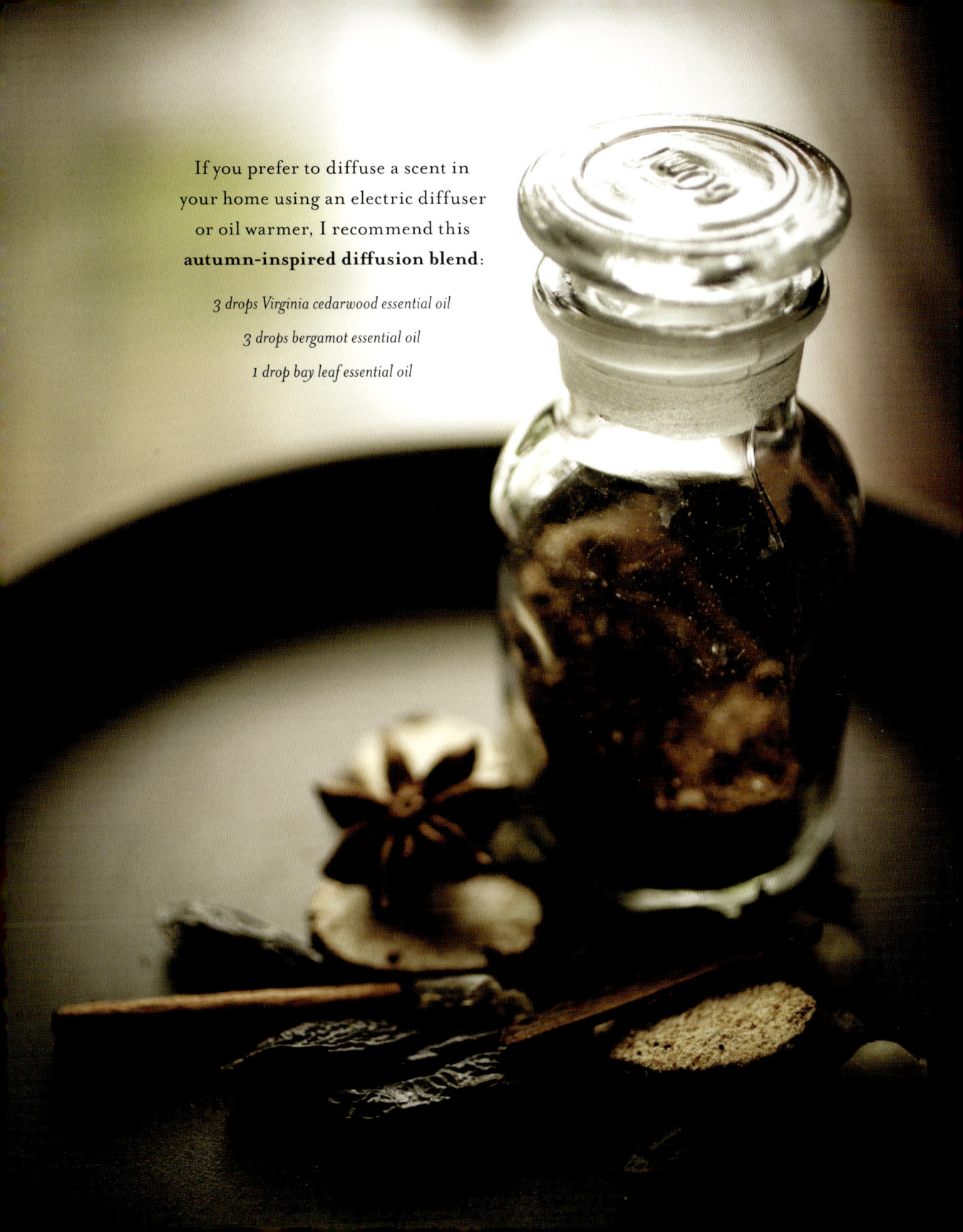

If you prefer to diffuse a scent in your home using an electric diffuser or oil warmer, I recommend this **autumn-inspired diffusion blend**:

3 drops Virginia cedarwood essential oil

3 drops bergamot essential oil

1 drop bay leaf essential oil

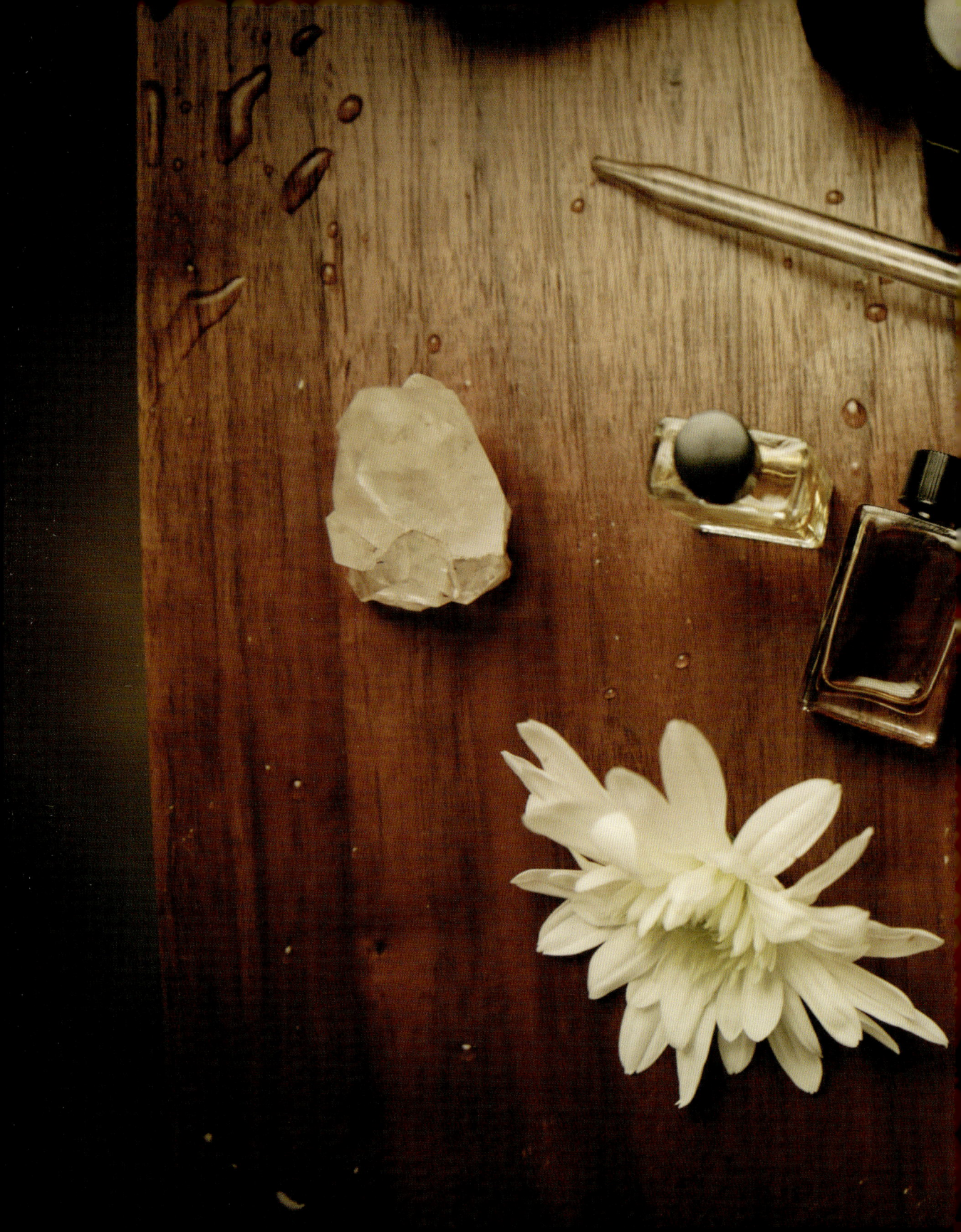

Winter

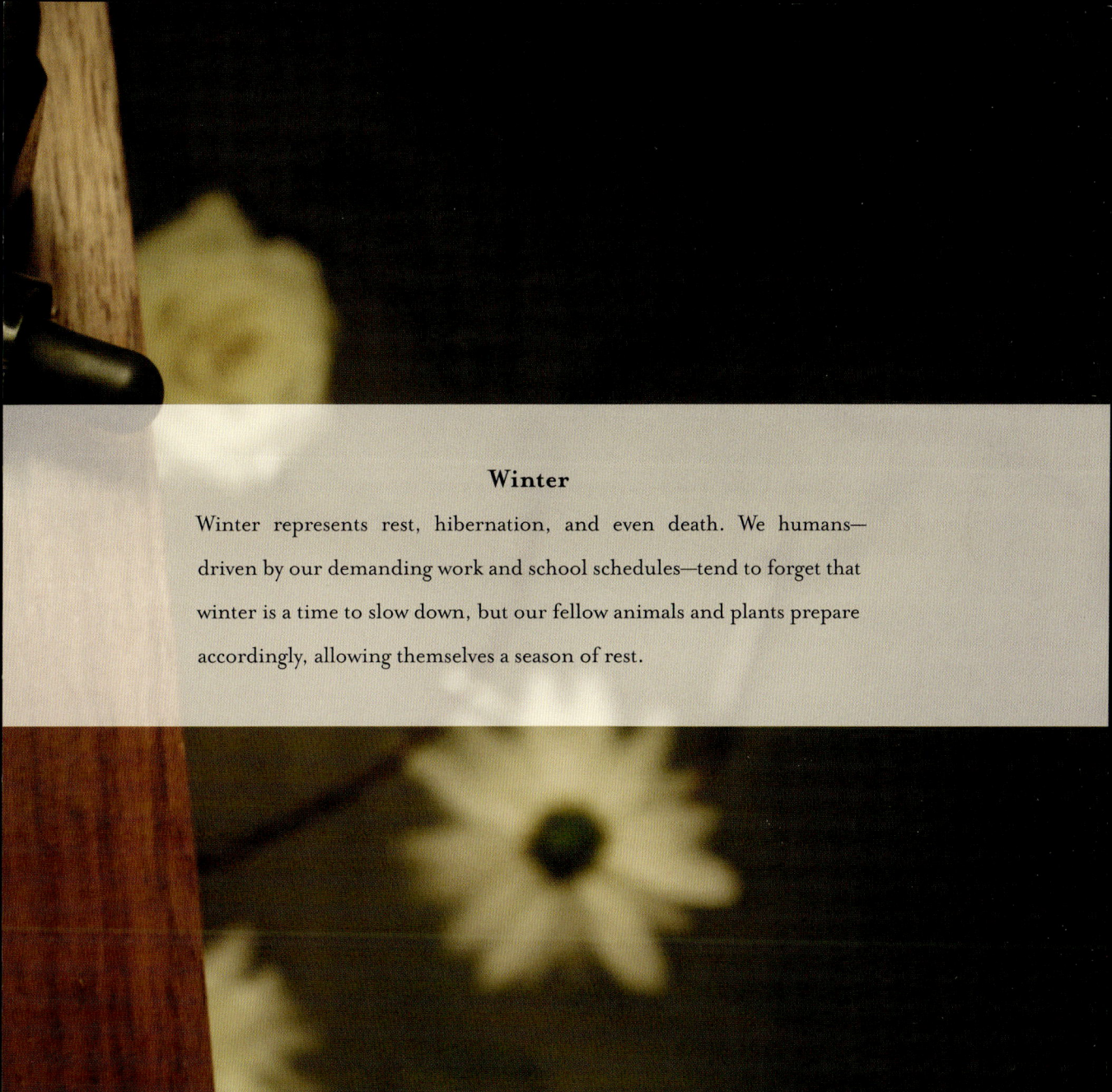

Winter represents rest, hibernation, and even death. We humans—driven by our demanding work and school schedules—tend to forget that winter is a time to slow down, but our fellow animals and plants prepare accordingly, allowing themselves a season of rest.

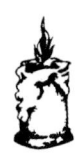

WINTER SOLSTICE RITUAL BATH

A ritual bath is perfect for a snowy day, and especially the winter solstice. Enjoy this bath as a way of honoring the shortest day of the year, relaxing along with the rest of the natural world.

6 green tea bags

1 12-ounce can full-fat coconut milk

7 drops fir needle essential oil

3 drops peppermint essential oil

1 cup Epsom salt (magnesium sulfate)

Foraged cedar leaves, or spruce or fir needles

If there is snow available outside your home, gather a large bowl of it and bring it inside; allow it to melt. If you don't have access to snow, simply fill a bowl with water.

Place your intentions into the water energetically. The idea is that the energy of your thoughts is transferred to the water in physical form. Simply imagine this happening.

Heat the water to a simmer and use it to brew the green tea in a French press; let it steep for three minutes.

Run a warm bath.

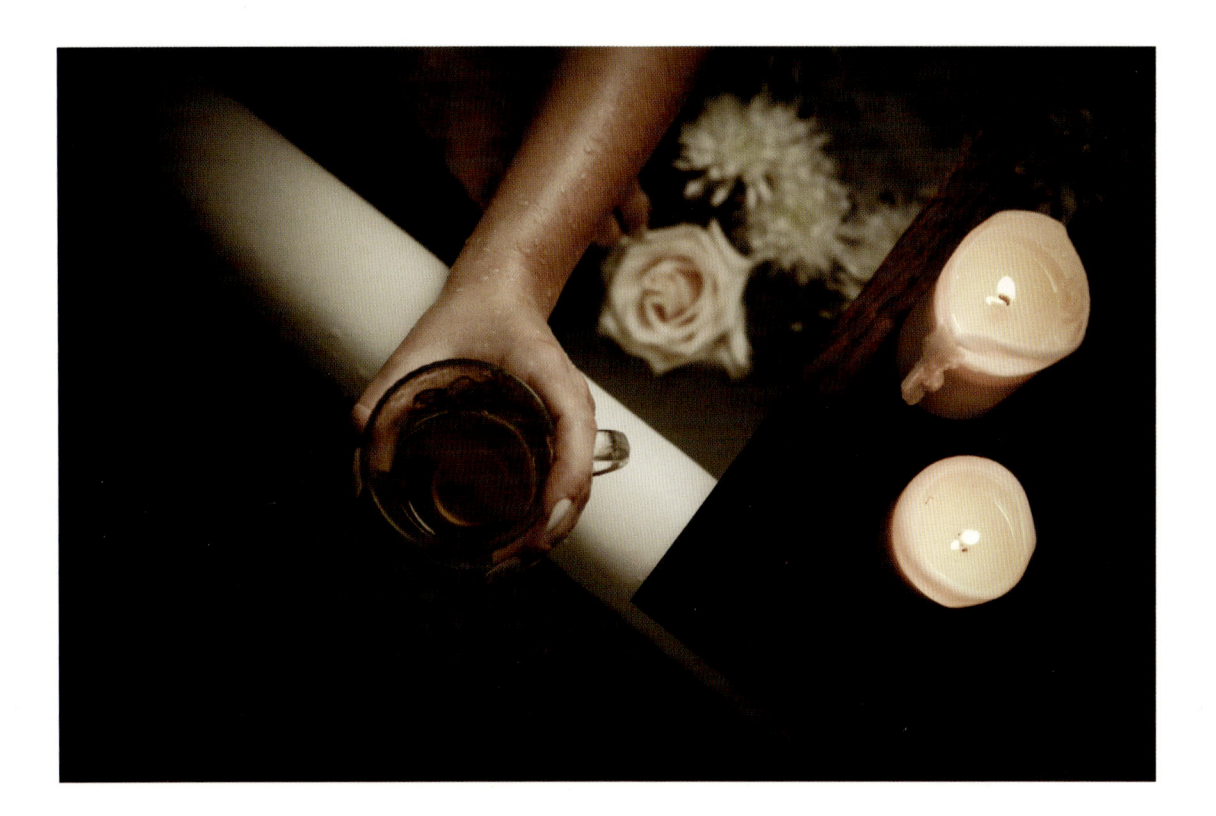

Pour the tea into the bathwater along with the coconut milk, fir needle and peppermint essential oils, Epsom salt, and foraged materials. Full-fat coconut milk is very moisturizing for dry winter skin. The oil in it also helps to disperse the essential oils.

Because the solstice is the longest night of the year, I recommend lighting unscented beeswax candles around this bath as a way of welcoming back the light, which begins to reappear after this night. Add any crystals, music, herbs, and incense you wish.

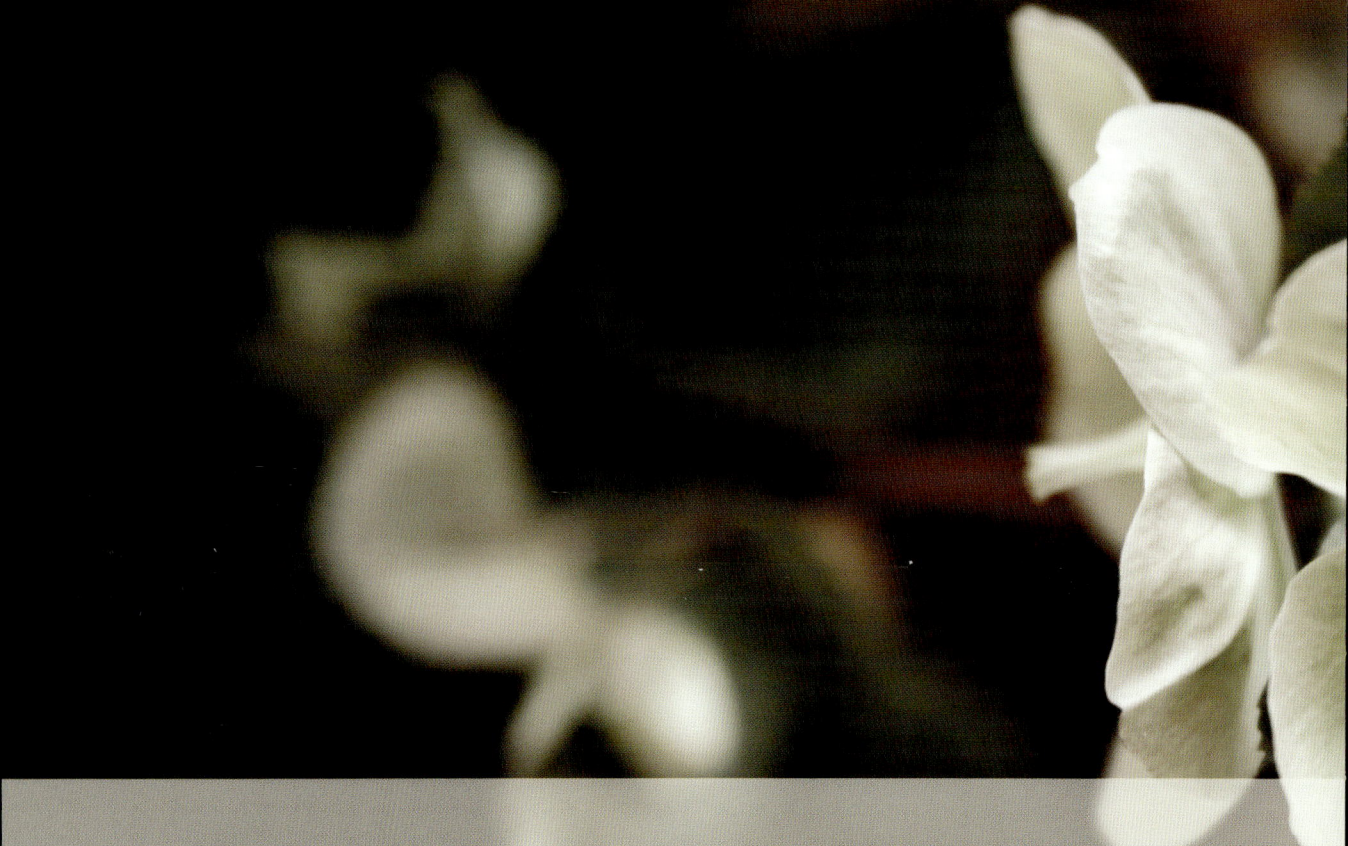

Spring

The equinoxes are my favorite times of the year because they bring balance. The day and night are even in length and the weather recovers from extremes. The spring equinox brings new growth and resurrection in nature, and we can harness this energy to begin new pursuits. It is a highly creative time, and with the increased sunlight, we naturally gain more energy.

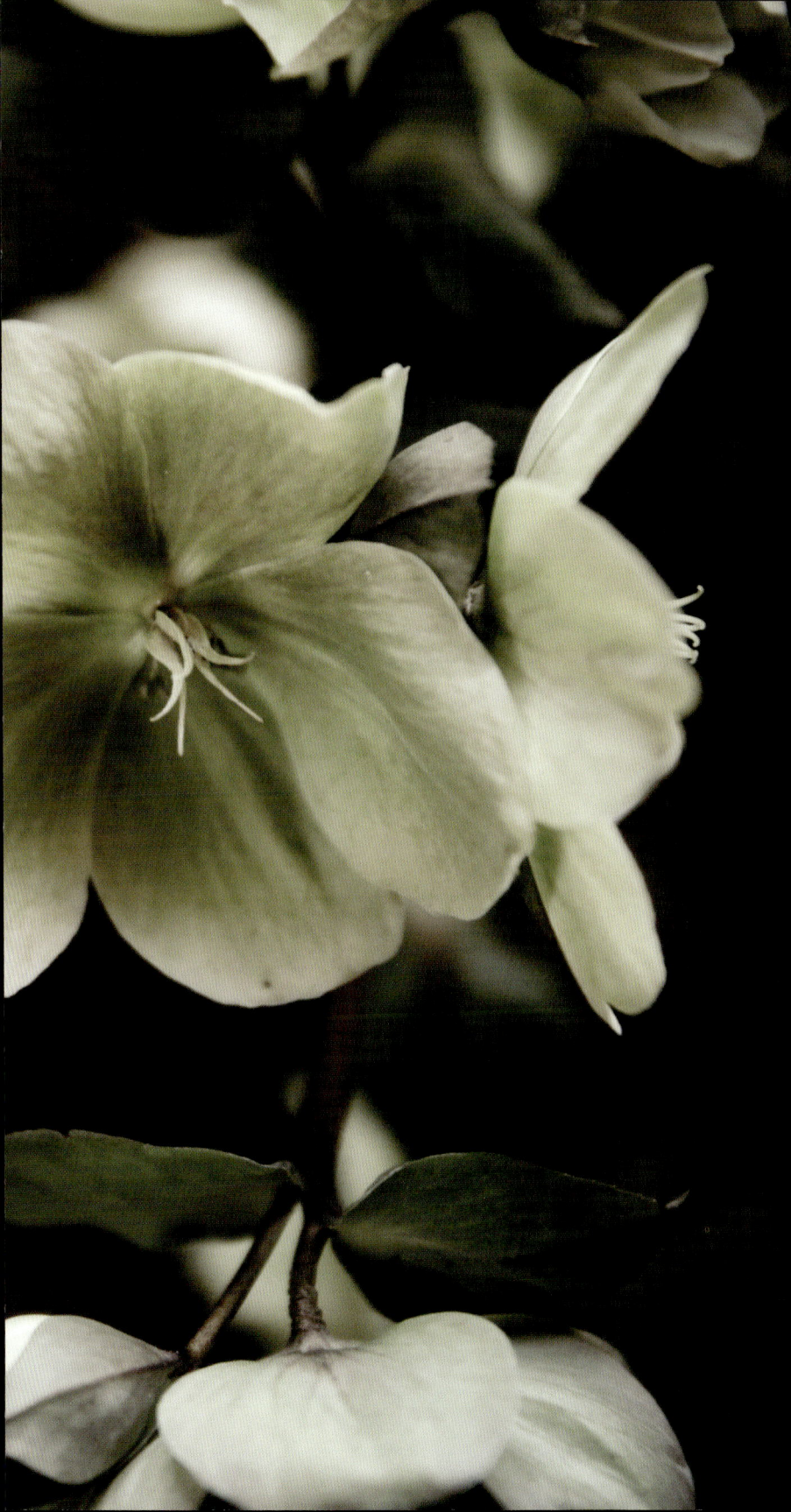

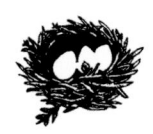

SPRING EQUINOX PERFUME

Makes 1 ounce

This perfume, which can also be used as a room or linen spray, features a tincture of propolis, a material that is made by honeybees from the resins they collect from trees and other plants. The bees combine the resins into a single substance they use to seal and protect their hives. It is a precious material that should be used sparingly; luckily, a little will go a long way. It may be difficult to source propolis, but many beekeepers sell a small amount from their hives.

PROPOLIS TINCTURE

½ teaspoon coarsely ground propolis resin

4 teaspoons (20 milliliters) organic 190-proof alcohol

PERFUME

12 milliliters lavender tincture (see page 49)

5 milliliters propolis tincture

6 drops frankincense essential oil

10 drops vetiver essential oil

12 milliliters rose water (organic rose hydrosol)

For the propolis tincture, combine the propolis resin and alcohol in a small glass jar (at least 2-ounce capacity) with an airtight lid and seal. Allow to tincture for 2 weeks. (You may notice that the propolis completely dissolves within 1 week.)

For the perfume, combine 12 milliliters of the lavender tincture and 5 milliliters of the propolis tincture in a 1-ounce glass bottle with a fine-mist sprayer, reserving any remaining tincture for another use. Add the frankincense and vetiver essential oils. Fill the rest of the bottle with the rose water. Screw on the top and shake to blend. Label and store in a cool, dark place.

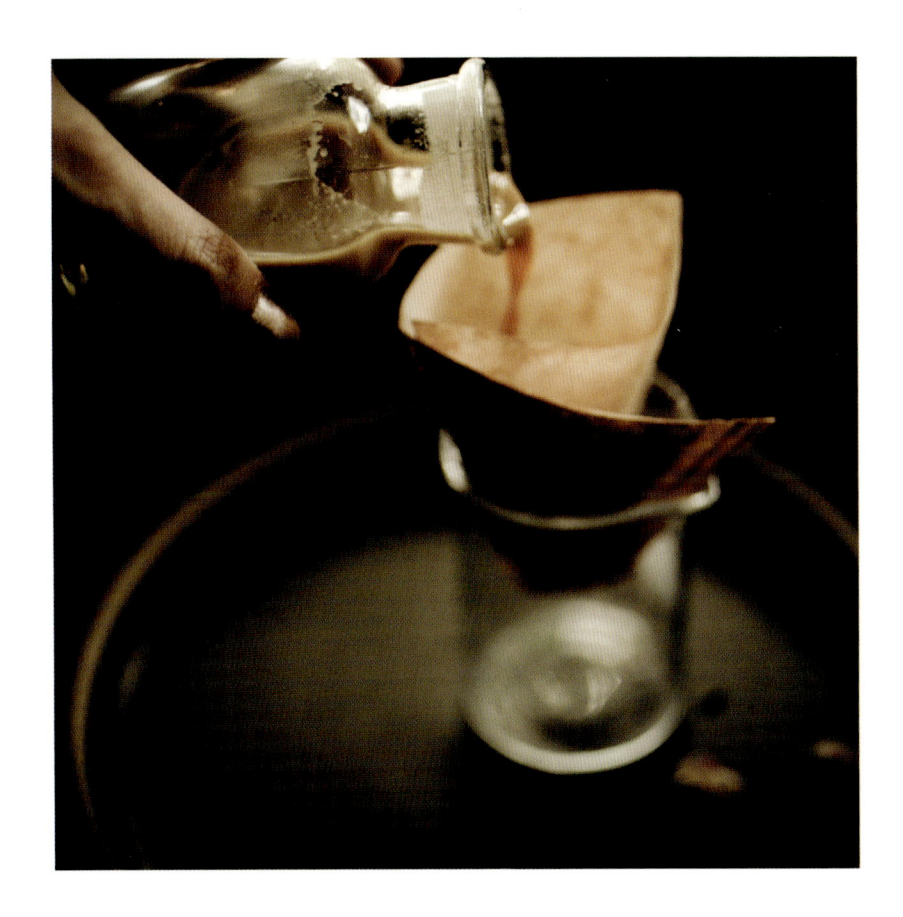

Summer

The summer solstice, also referred to as midsummer, is the longest day of the year and an important celebration in pagan cultures. The ancient Celts, my ancestors, were believed to celebrate with parties and bonfires, so this is my chosen tradition. The summer heat can be intense in my region, so I complement the fire with cooling garden tisanes.

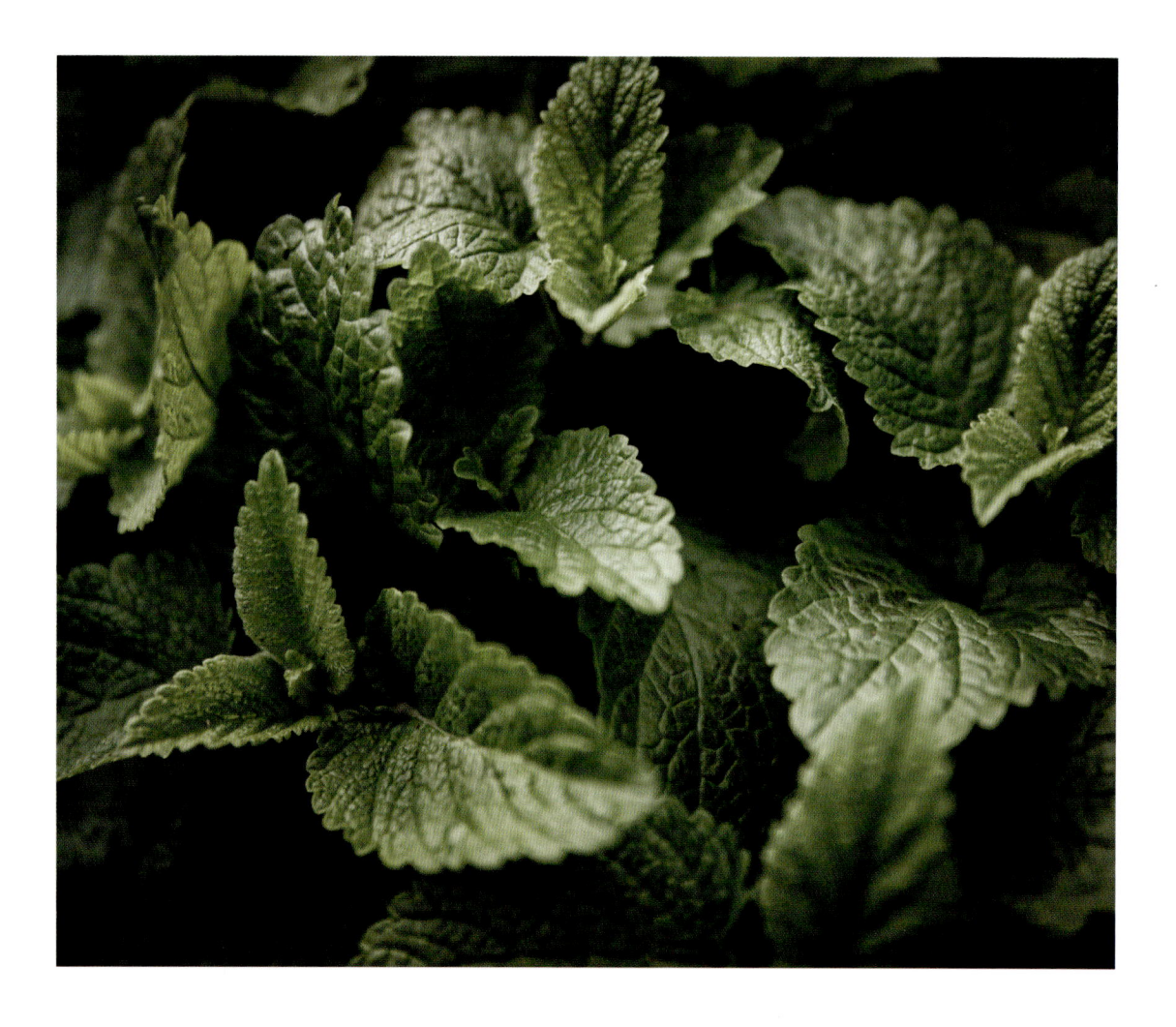

MIDSUMMER ICED MINT TISANE

Serves 3 to 4

It's best to use fresh herbs for this tea, which tend to be more cooling to our blood than dried herbs. To balance the long days and heat of the summer, I rely on the mint family. I grow beds of chocolate-scented peppermint, lemon balm, and tulsi (also known as holy basil) in my backyard, so I have a continuous supply of the herbs used in this calming tea. In my region, these are all very easy plants to grow, and if in the ground, they spread quickly. Sometimes I add in other fresh materials from the garden, including strawberry and blackberry leaves, borage flowers, and chamomile. At the solstice, plants have more of the sun's energy than at any other time, and an early morning harvest ensures the strongest scent.

Fresh lemon balm, rinsed with stems removed
Peppermint, rinsed with stems removed
Tulsi, rinsed with stems removed
Sweetener, if desired

Place a fully packed cup of the fresh herb leaves into a French press and fill with hot water. Add the sweetener if using. Allow the infusion to steep for 10 to 20 minutes, then place it in the refrigerator overnight.

The next day, press to filter the leaves, and enjoy the tisane over ice.

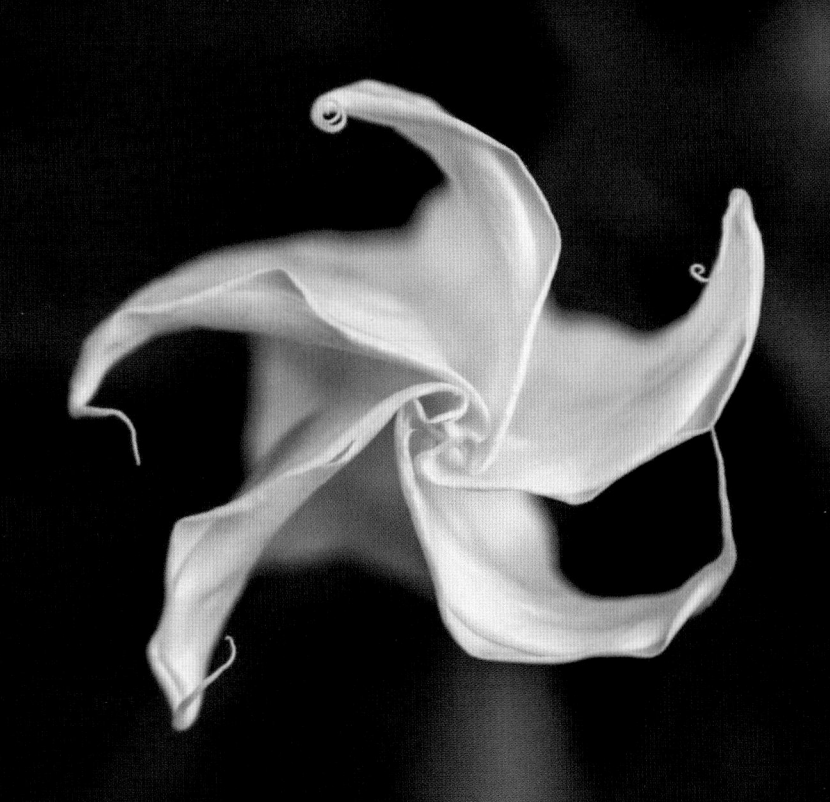

Eight

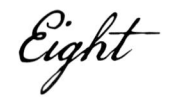

THE MOON

When I began For Strange Women, I had trouble adjusting to working for myself. I didn't know how to balance my time and energy with work and deadlines. I needed to establish a more sustainable pace and schedule to avoid burnout. My zodiac sign is Cancer, which is ruled by the moon, so I began working with her energy to balance my own. As my energy synchronized with the moon's cycles, I established a more natural pace for work, rest, initiation, harvest, completion, and organization.

We know that the moon's gravitational force pulls on the water in the ground and oceans. On a more subtle level, it also pulls on the water within our bodies. Since we are about 60 percent water, there are certain biodynamic practices that can help us work with our inner tides.

New Moon/ Waxing Crescent

When the moon goes dark, it has reached the same side of the earth as the sun. On the first day of the new moon, it's important to focus on the intentions and goals you have for this moon cycle. This is an ideal time for reflection, slowing down, and meditating or journaling. From this new beginning until the waxing crescent reaches the first quarter, the moon supports the development of new projects.

First Quarter/ Waxing Gibbous

As the half moon grows toward the full moon, we experience a time of increased momentum and growth. You may feel the most challenged during this time as the weight of the full moon presses in. Problem-solving and flexibility are important at this time, as difficult decisions may arise.

Full Moon

The opposing pulls from the sun and moon on either side of the earth coupled with the brighter sky at night can amplify anything that happens. The full moon is a time to harness this extra energy to communicate, to harvest, or to add intensity to a message or event. The added light can illuminate things that were previously hidden, and emotions are often intensified. It is recommended to create intentions of release at this time, in hopes that unwanted aspects of our lives will disappear along with the moon's light over the next two weeks.

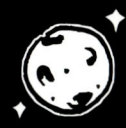

FULL MOON BOTANICAL TRANCE OIL

Makes about 5 milliliters

3½ milliliters (about 100 drops) jojoba oil

17 drops clary sage essential oil

9 drops neroli essential oil (also called orange blossom essential oil)

7 drops lavender essential oil

Combine all ingredients in a 5-milliliter glass bottle with an airtight lid and seal. Store in a cool, dark place.

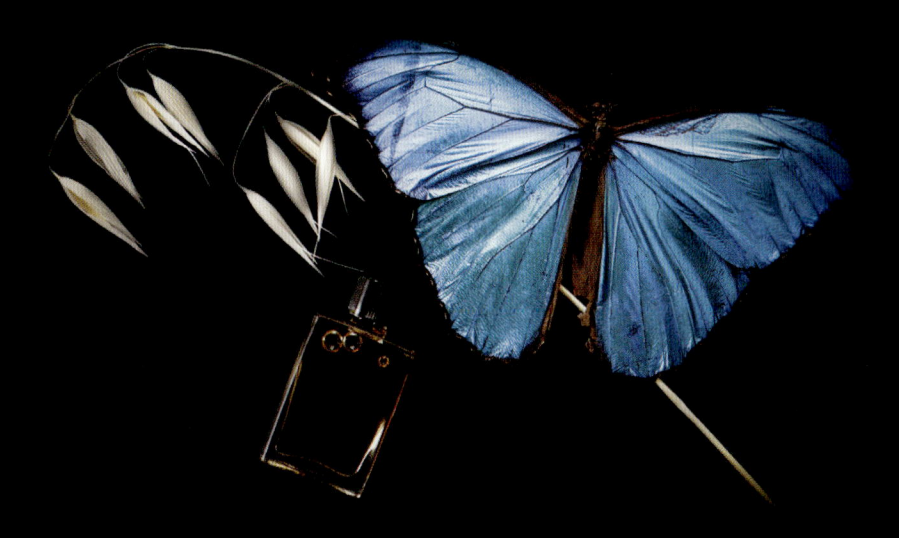

Full Moon Guided Trance

Ask a partner to guide you through the following text by reading it aloud to you while you lie down in a quiet place without any other distractions. Your partner should be sitting close behind or beside you. Make sure the temperature and lighting in the space are comfortable for you and that you are in a position that feels supported. Apply a small amount of the **Full Moon Botanical Trance Oil** to your neck and wrists, focusing on the scent as you inhale deeply. Listen closely as your partner reads the following instructions to you.

Apply this oil to your wrists and neck. As you settle into a comfortable position, let your eyes close, and prepare to be guided through five slow, deep breaths.

Inhale deeply, allowing the spirits of orange blossom, lavender, and clary sage to fill your lungs and your head. As you exhale slowly, recognize how peaceful, comfortable, and supported you feel.

Breathe in and notice how this essence has a color. . . . Breathe out and describe what color it is.

(Wait for Answer)

Breathe in this [color] energy and allow it to fill your lungs and head and then spread through the rest of your body. Exhale everything inside you that does not match this color.

Breathe in and notice the soft layers of the [color] scent, and as you exhale, notice how your blood carries the [color] molecules to every capillary and every cell of your body.

Breathe in and feel how every cell affected by this [color] scent is nourished, relaxed, and restructured. Notice that the anxiety you felt before is pushed out of your lungs as you exhale.

Continue to breathe normally and allow these botanical essences to guide you. Notice what images come to your mind and what messages you hear. Take a few minutes to follow these thoughts as they are guided by these plant spirits and the full moon's illumination. When you have found a place of completion, signal to me with your hand.

(Allow them to concentrate while you sit with them. Match your breathing to theirs and try to stay focused on them. When they signal to you, continue.)

As the full moon illuminates what is usually dark, use this light to see into places of your life that you were unable to see before. You are supported by the moon and the earth and all the spirits of nature. As I ask the following questions, take your time to allow the answers to find you. You can tell me what you notice or just think to yourself. When you are ready to move on, signal to me with your hand.

What has this [color] energy done to transform your mind and your spirit?

What has this [color] energy done to transform your physical body?

What is this full moon illuminating about your current life?

Thank you to the orange blossom, the lavender, and the clary sage for their guidance. Take another deep breath, and feel a return to the surface of your awareness. Move your fingers . . . your toes . . . and whenever you are ready, open your eyes.

Last Quarter

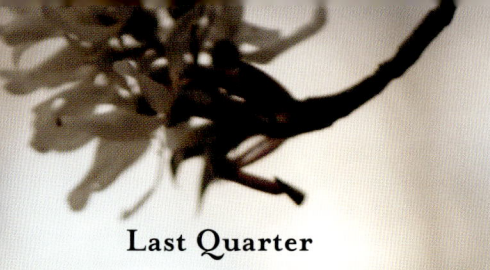

As the last quarter of the moon wanes to the new moon, the emotions, ideas, and creations stirred up by the full moon have a chance to settle. It is best, at this time, to let go of the critical decision-making mindset you inhabited during the first quarter and to relax, allowing any open projects or communications to find closure. Tie up loose ends, clean, organize, and prepare for the new moon during this phase. Clear away anything that clutters your mind and space so that you are able to start over with a clean slate. This way, when the new moon arrives, its flood of creative, emotional, and inspirational energy can move through you without interference.

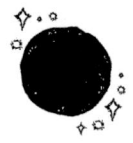

NEW MOON CLEANING INFUSION

Makes 16 ounces

During the growing season, I gather herbs from my garden and infuse them in white vinegar to create cleaning supplies. Throughout the year, in the last days of the waning crescent, I clean my house to prepare for each new moon. This is an all-purpose surface cleaner that is so much safer and more satisfying to use than commercial chemical sprays. Since most household cleaners are indoor air contaminants, I have always preferred to create my own nontoxic cleaners that contain the plant spirits of my garden. Thyme and oregano are two herbs with powerful antimicrobial properties. You might also consider adding fresh rosemary, sage, parsley, basil, and/or lavender.

Fresh herbs of choice
1⅛ cup distilled white vinegar
1 cup distilled water

Add the fresh herbs to a 16-ounce mason jar, filling to the top. Pour in the vinegar, covering the herbs completely. Seal the lid tightly and allow to infuse for 4 weeks (one moon cycle). Using a fine-mesh strainer or cheesecloth, strain the infused vinegar into a container; discard the herbs. Using a funnel, fill a 16-ounce glass spray bottle with 1 cup of the vinegar infusion and the distilled water. Screw on the top and shake to blend. Store in a cool, dark place. Another option: Combine ½ cup of infused vinegar with 1 gallon of hot water to use as a floor cleaner.

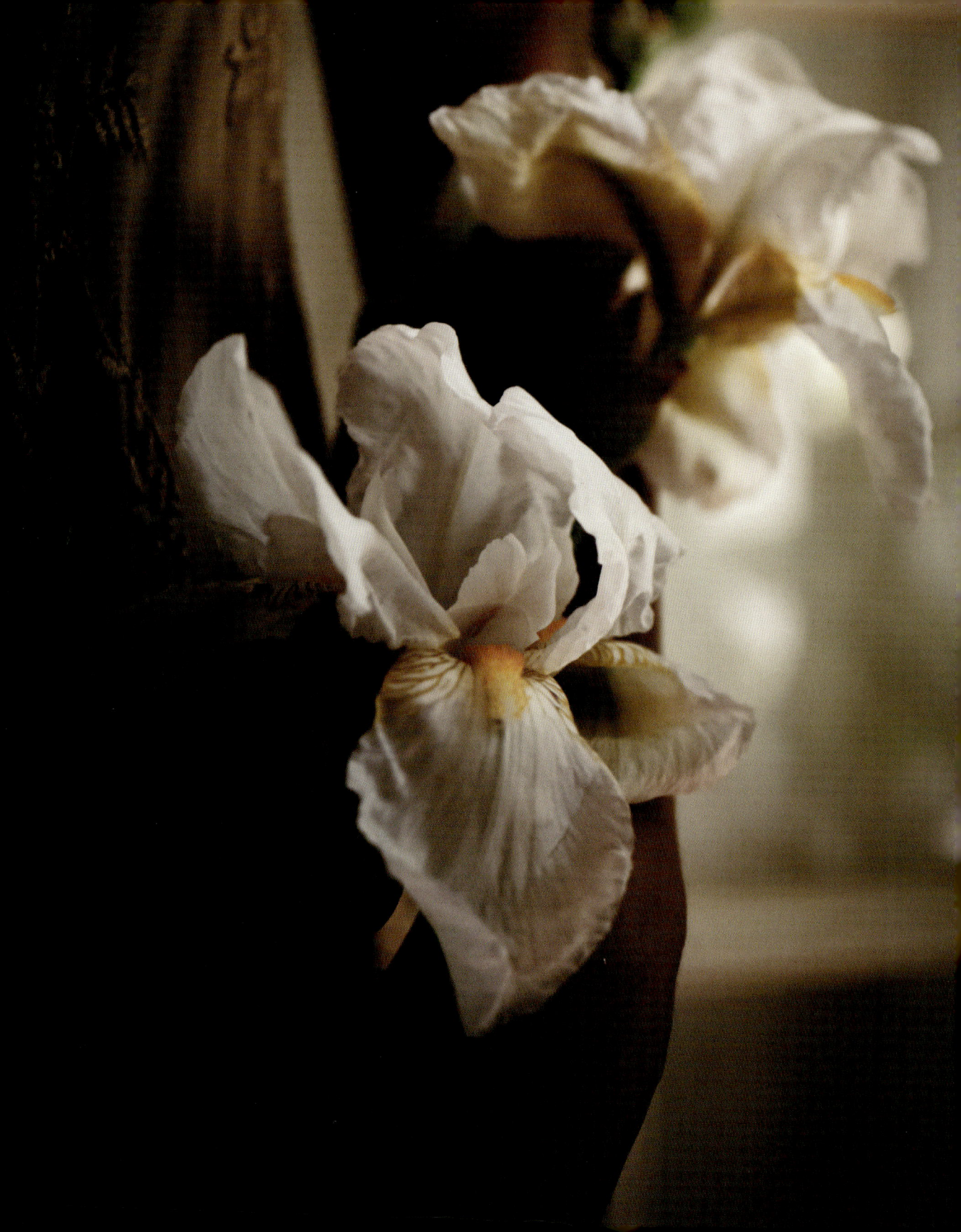

Nine

AROMATHERAPY

Scent and the Mind

I am often asked which of my perfumes will help most with anxiety and depression. Everyone has to deal with these states to some extent, and some are debilitated by them. Given the corrupt state of our pharmaceutical industry and the sometimes devastating side effects of synthetic drugs, it doesn't surprise me that so many people are looking for natural ways to address their mental health concerns.

I have found the following blend combined with a breathing meditation (or simply an effort to deepen my breath) to be very helpful in relieving anxiety.

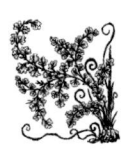

ANTI-ANXIETY AROMATHERAPY INHALER

4 drops Australian sandalwood essential oil

3 drops fir essential oil

2 drops cypress essential oil

1 drop eucalyptus essential oil

Fill a lip balm tube with a cotton ball or other absorbent natural fiber. Add the Australian sandalwood, fir, cypress, and eucalyptus essential oils to the cotton.

To use, throughout the day as needed, or during meditation, remove the lip balm tube lid and hold the tube below your nose, inhaling deeply. This inhaler will last at least several months and up to a year if stored in a cool, dark place.

You can also use this blend in an aromatherapy diffuser or by using the HVAC diffusion method (see "Home Integrations," page 104).

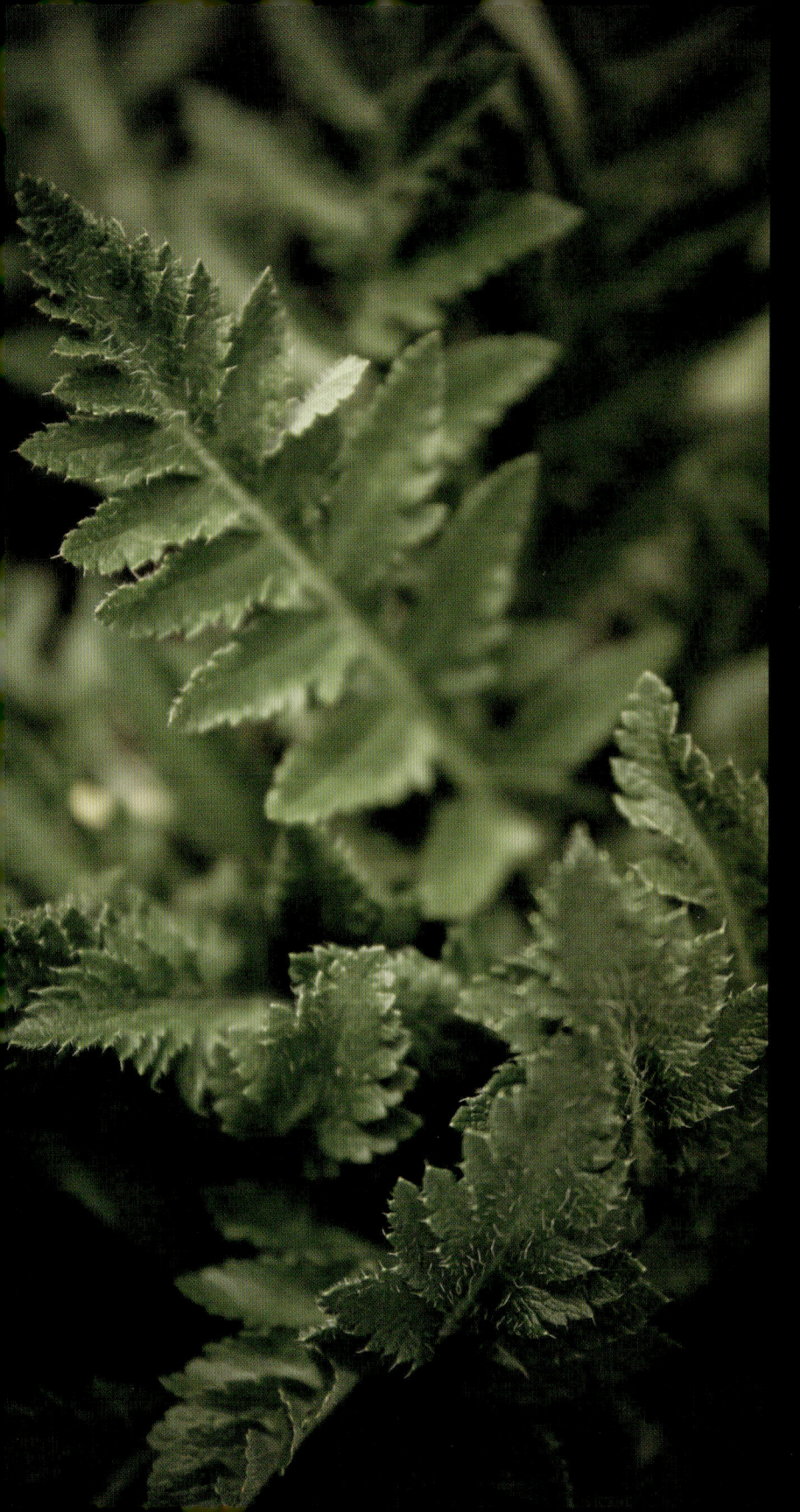

Anxiety often causes me to forget to inhale or to take only shallow breaths. During a trip to Japan, I noticed that I began to breathe more deeply when I entered a Buddhist temple, where the air was delicately scented with a gorgeous blend of sandalwood and agarwood. The subtlety of the scent was similar to the whisper of natural perfume as it dries down on the skin. Inhaling the wood essences, I consumed their messages. The incense made me more conscious of the air and the way I interacted with it, naturally guiding me into a meditation.

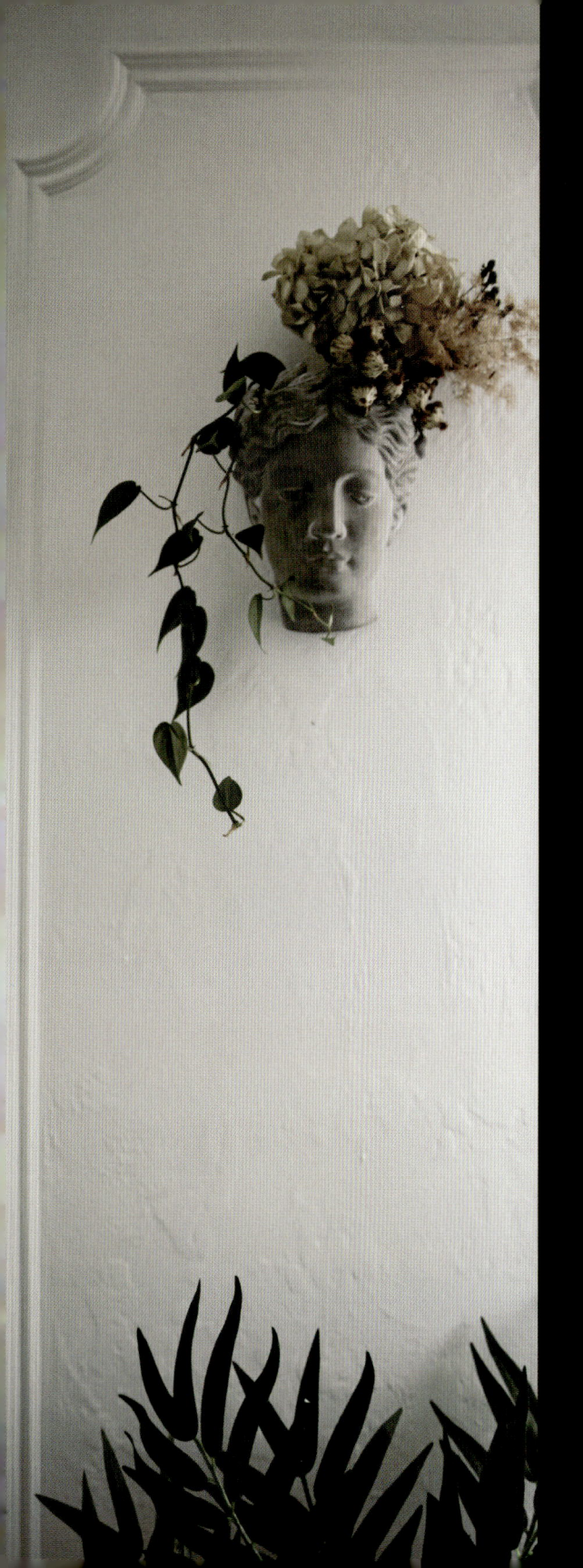

Home Integrations

- If you're able to source hydrosols and want to find more uses for them, there are many creative ways to cook using them (or brewed teas or tisanes) in place of water. Try replacing the water in recipes for breads, cookies, cakes, and other baked goods with rose or orange blossom water.

- Most houses have an HVAC system, which I consider to be the perfect aromatherapy diffuser. When I want to circulate a scent in my home, I remove the filter, put a couple of drops of essential oil on it, and put it back in place. Then I turn on the fan to circulate the scent throughout the house. (Note: Eucalyptus and peppermint oils are stimulating and clean, but these scents can bother pets. For use in homes with pets, I suggest more animal-friendly notes, such as jasmine, lavender, Australian sandalwood, and clary sage.)

- I use unscented soaps and laundry detergent in my home, but sometimes I like to add a natural scent to laundry. When I machine-dry towels and sheets, I add a few drops of essential oil to wool dryer balls. My favorite oil to use for a clean scent is eucalyptus, but I also love fir, sage, and rosemary. Be sure to run your dryer on medium or low heat, as high heat will weaken the scent.

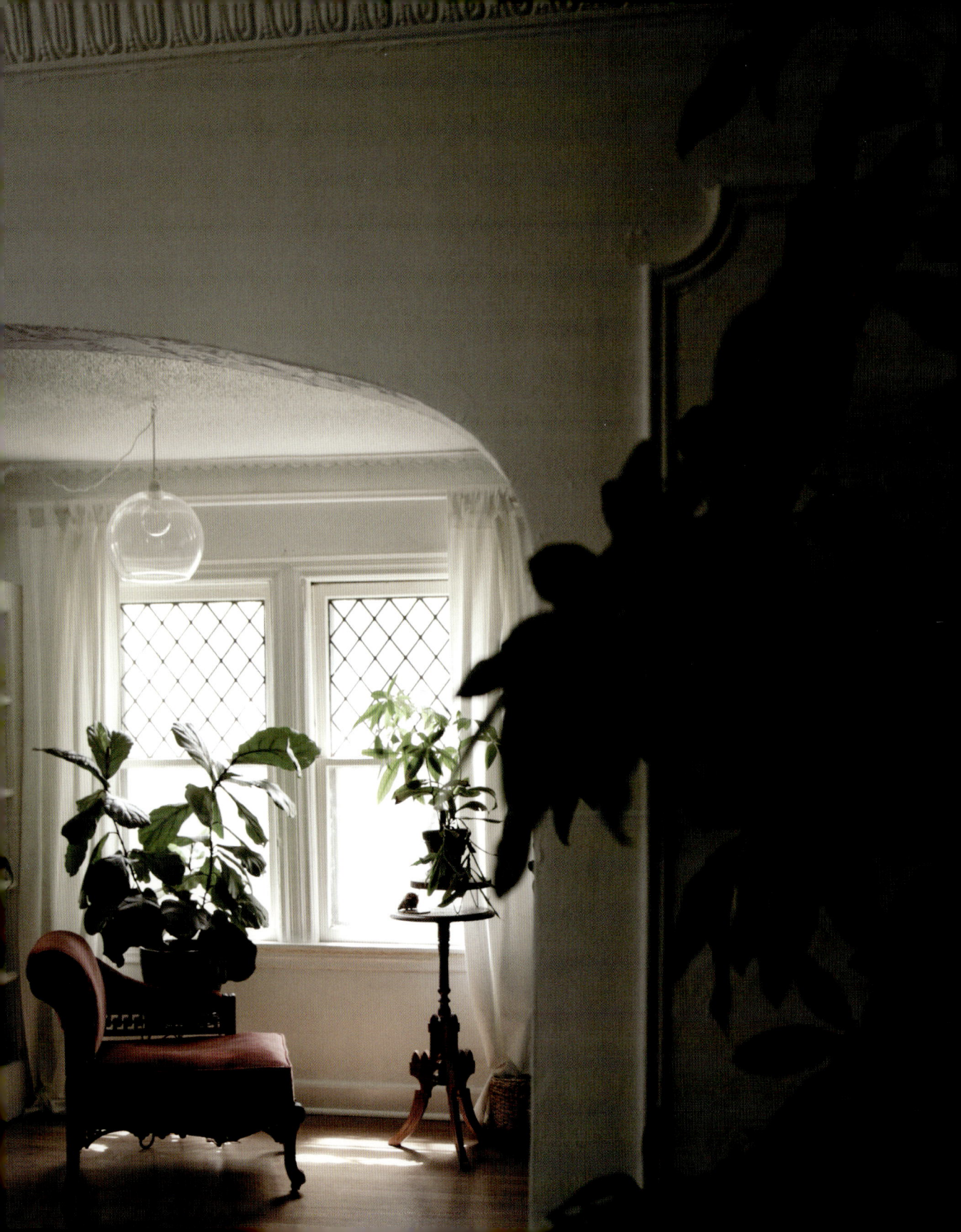

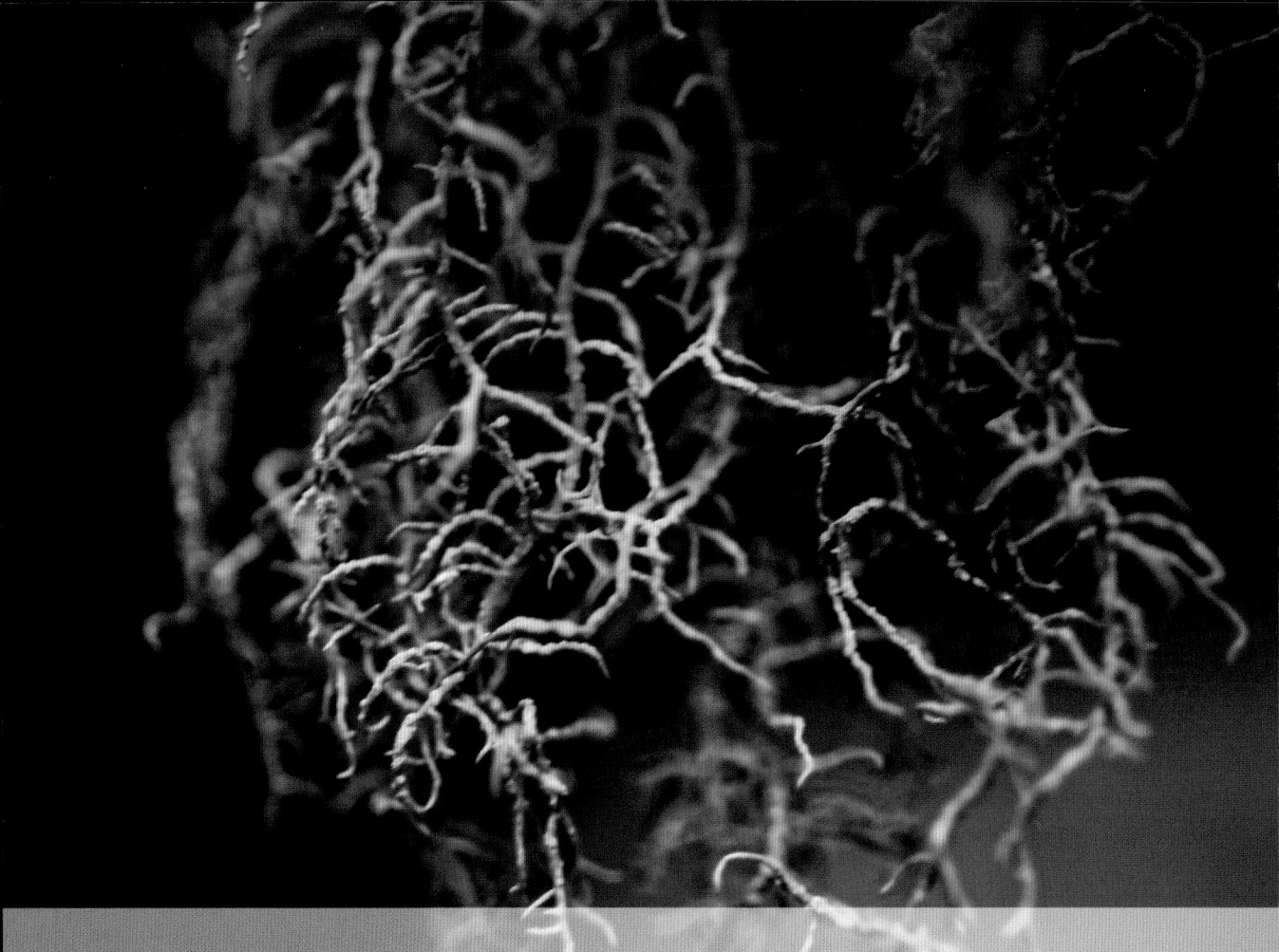

More Aromatherapy Blends

Aromatherapy is second only to music in its ability to quickly change my state of mind. These plant essences (from the plant or from their extracted essential oils) are helpful for inducing a number of different mental and emotional states. Combine several of them to make your own blend, or use one note on its own. These can be used in a diffuser, an aromatherapy inhaler, or even as a personal blend to wear when diluted to 2 to 10 percent with a carrier oil. It is also effective to smell them directly from the bottle, consuming no more than what evaporates when you remove the lid.

relax: lavender, neroli, rose, tulsi, sandalwood, bergamot

wake up: palo santo, grapefruit, *may chang*, peppermint, eucalyptus

sleep: lavender, valerian, chamomile, hops

create: orange, sandalwood, patchouli, ylang-ylang, sweet basil

meditate: Use single notes for meditation. My favorite is Australian sandalwood.

seduce: jasmine, vanilla, frankincense, orris root

travel: peppermint, ginger

memory: rosemary, sage

Geographical Scentscapes

Another way of categorizing scent is by landscape. Do you love the beach, or do you feel most at home in the forest? Perhaps you wish to revisit an important memory or feeling that took place in a certain topography. Aromatherapy is a way to travel, visiting the landscapes that heal you, without ever leaving your home.

MOUNTAINS

For me, the mountains are where I feel most protected and safe. I first visited the mountains on a trip to Colorado when I was sixteen. I was listening to Rasputina's *Thanks for the Ether* CD on repeat the entire trip. Now, when I want to connect with the mountains from a distance, I listen to that album and burn an incense blend that returns me to the place where I felt most at home.

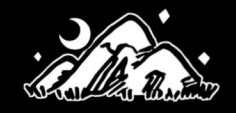

MOUNTAIN INCENSE

Makes ⅛ cup of loose incense (or 12 uses)

---

*1 teaspoon fresh pine needles, cut into ½-inch pieces
(these are fun and easy to forage)*

1 teaspoon dried lavender buds

1 teaspoon crushed tree resin (white copal, benzoin, or frankincense)

1 teaspoon orris root powder

1 teaspoon dried sweetgrass, cut into ½-inch pieces

1 teaspoon sandalwood powder or white oak bark powder (optional)

Combine all of the ingredients and place half a teaspoon of the mixture on bamboo charcoal to burn as incense (see "How to Burn Loose Incense," page 71).

This blend may also be tinctured, filtered, and used as a room or linen spray (see "How to Tincture," page 8). Just be sure to leave out the resin if storing in a spray bottle.

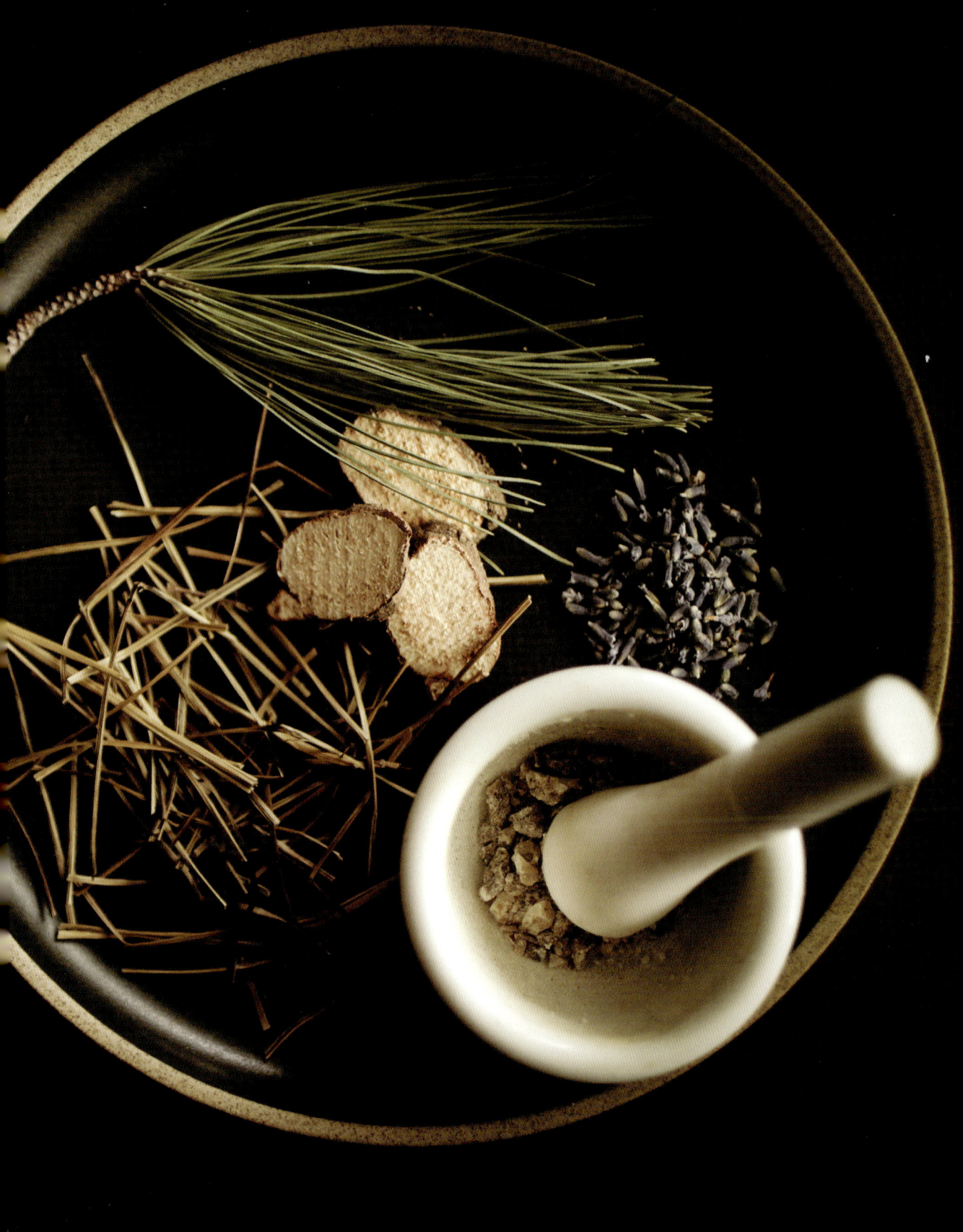

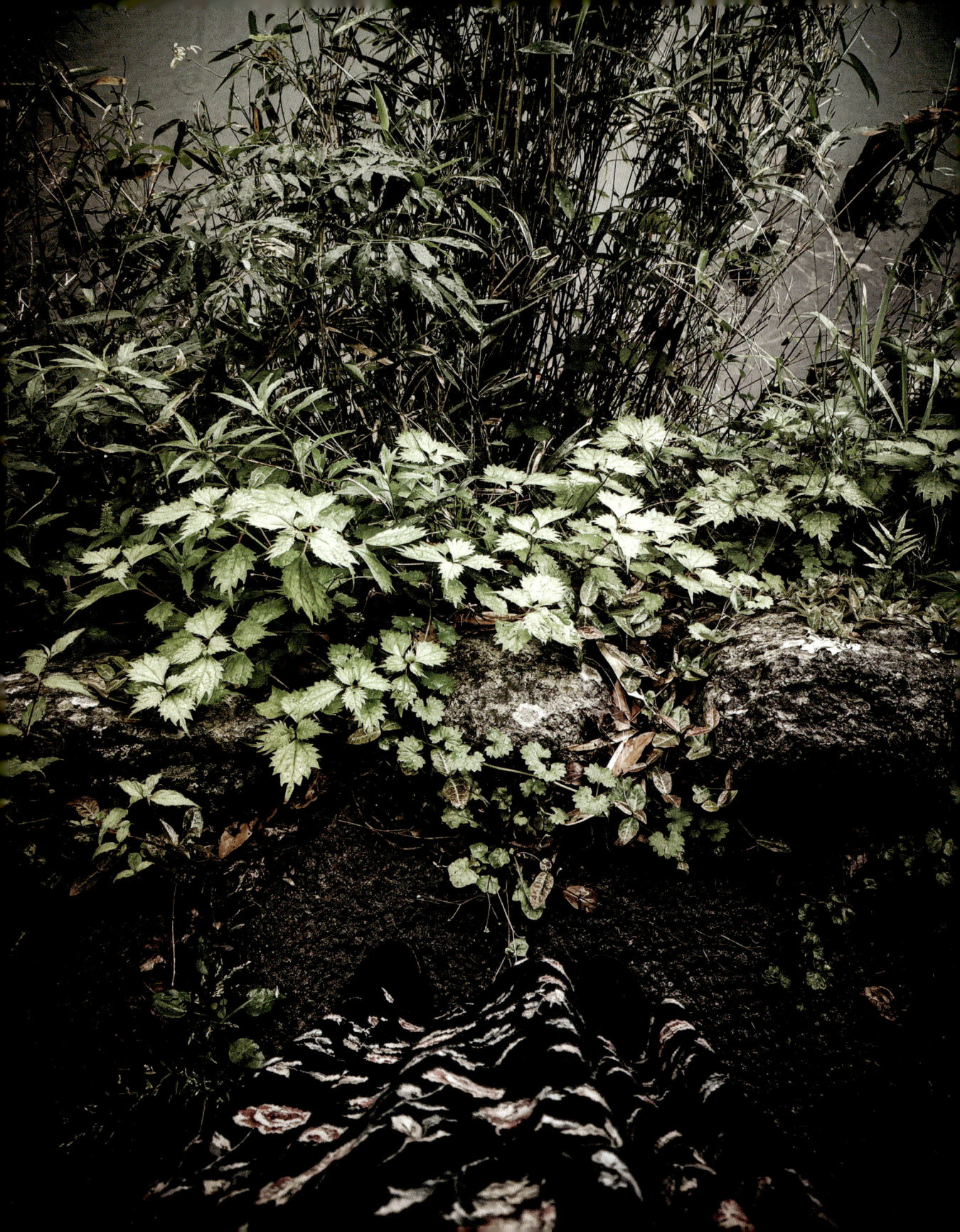

OCEAN

The first tincture in this book, the **Tincture for Strange Women** (see page 6), is an ocean tincture. The kombu mixed with fresh jasmine, rosemary, and lavender evokes a northern coastal landscape. Other materials that can be tinctured to conjure an ocean scent are lime peels, seashells, and other dried sea vegetables.

DESERT

The **Incense Blend for Spirit Cleansing, Protection, and Strength** (see page 75) re-creates the dry atmosphere and botanical elements of the desert. Frankincense, myrrh, and piñon resins are also ideal for invoking the energy of the desert. Burn these over charcoal.

TEMPERATE DECIDUOUS FOREST

There are many different types of forests, but the temperate deciduous is my home. This forest undergoes a cycle of new life and decomposition throughout the year. The standing woods and foliage have a light, fresh scent that is deepened by a floor of moss, lichen, mushrooms, and fallen tree matter. To bring these scents into my home, I sometimes add fallen dried leaves from my sycamore tree to my incense blends. I also wear perfumes with a base of oakmoss and woods and drink *pu-erh* tea, which is a fermented and aged tea from the Yunnan province of China with an earthy, complex flavor that reminds me of the forest floor.

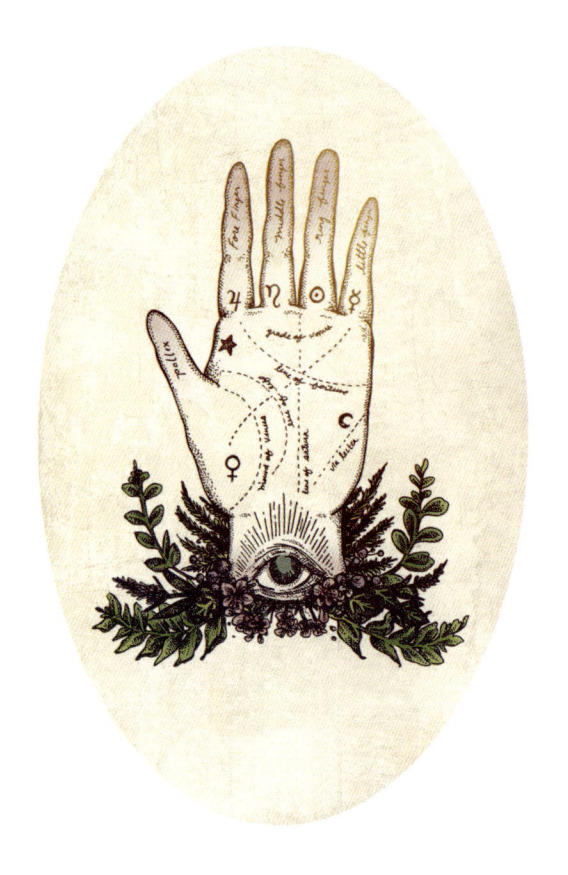

Scent and Astrology

I have a habit of noticing the astrological influences at work in those close to me, and I like to incorporate these observations into the custom perfumes I create. I pay attention to the aromatics people are drawn to and look for patterns in their chart dynamics. Below are some of the scent "horoscopes" I have developed as a result. Depending on your full astrological chart, you may identify with a mixture of these influences; these observations generally correspond to the sun signs.

ARIES *(March 21–April 19)*

You may gravitate toward scents that contain warm spices, energetic citrus, and a bold, commanding presence. Does it draw attention to you? Even better. Still, it would be beneficial for you to experiment with scents of a softer nature—soft florals, lavender, and resins—to temper your fiery nature.

TAURUS *(April 20–May 20)*

Your scent direction is very similar to that of a Libra, only with more culinary elements. You tend toward the simpler, more elegant blends and prefer sweet and clean notes over musky, dirty ones. Because you are the most sensual of the earth signs, you have more of an appreciation for soft balsams, resins, and fleshy florals.

GEMINI *(May 21–June 21)*

You can never settle on what you want to be from one day to the next, so why not have several totally different perfumes to match your multiple personalities? You will feel the urge to layer them indiscriminately, but I strongly caution you against that—if you are planning to leave the house.

──── **CANCER** (*June 22–July 22*) ────

Can a perfume offer you emotional support? I certainly hope so. You may need lots of citrus, eucalyptus, and evergreen needles to lift you up one day, and cocoa and sandalwood to comfort you the next. You may become obsessed with one perfume for several weeks, then move on to another—and you're not afraid of the dark and smoky scents, either.

──── **LEO** (*July 23–August 22*) ────

There's no stopping you, so you may as well go for those bold, sexy, look-at-me scents that attract you. Heady florals like jasmine and gardenia, energetic citrus notes, and other head turners like tobacco and ginger match your contagious energy.

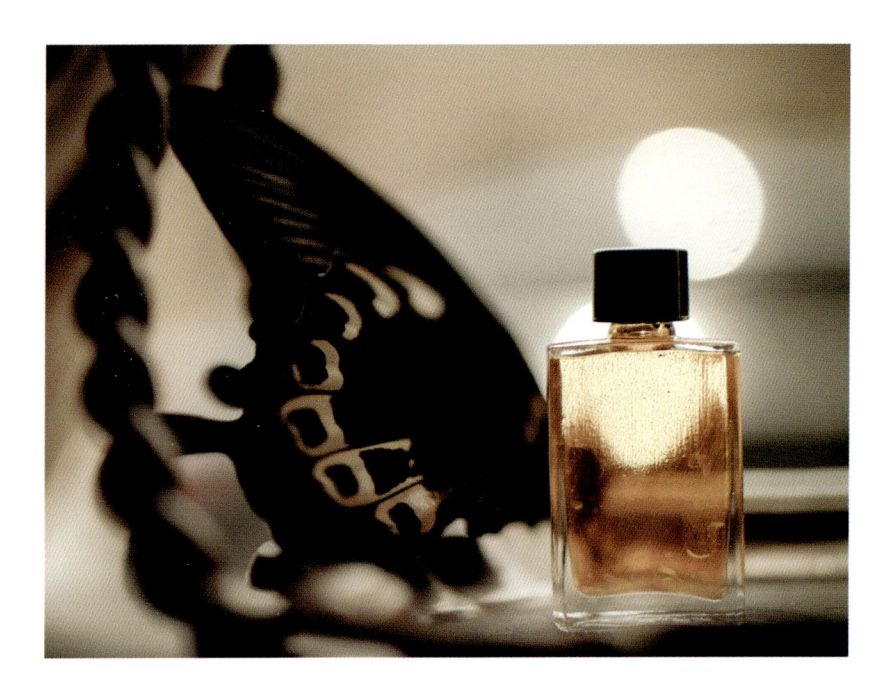

VIRGO (August 23–September 22)

You may have the strangest scent preferences of all. Your earthy nature craves musky root and wood scents, and a little patchouli never scared you. Anything that takes you out of your mind and into the present moment is great for you, so explore the rare notes—agarwood, lotus, and palo santo—to their fullest.

LIBRA (September 23–October 23)

An appreciator of fine aesthetics, you love deep florals—especially rose. You tend to like simple blends with clean scents balanced by sultry base notes like sandalwood or orris. You tend to be very particular, but when you settle on your favorite scent, it may never change.

SCORPIO (October 24–November 21)

You love scents that keep you in touch with your dark, mysterious self. You have no fear of androgynous perfumes, and you certainly don't care what anyone else thinks of your scent preference. Notes of leather, smoke, jasmine, and dark amber are especially appealing.

SAGITTARIUS (November 22–December 21)

Scent is perfectly tied to your sense of spirituality. From resins like frankincense and myrrh to aromatic woods, you are a lover of incense. A smoky undertone re-creates the incense smoke that surrounds you when you meditate.

CAPRICORN (December 22–January 19)

You know exactly what you like, and it's not sweet or fruity. The more sophisticated and refined scents are best for you, and you often have expensive taste. Oakmoss, lavender, rose, and other stress-reducing, relaxing scents are best for you.

AQUARIUS (January 20–February 18)

You're attracted to scents that remind you of another time or place. From fresh mountain air notes to spices that transport you to an open market in the Mediterranean, your favorite perfumes evoke your favorite places, historical events, and anthropological references.

PISCES (February 19–March 20)

You are sensitive enough to appreciate the subtler perfumes, and you gravitate toward comfort. Copaiba balsam, vanilla, sweet amber, and watery notes are like a warm hug in the form of a scent. Some woods blended in will offer the sense of stability you seek.

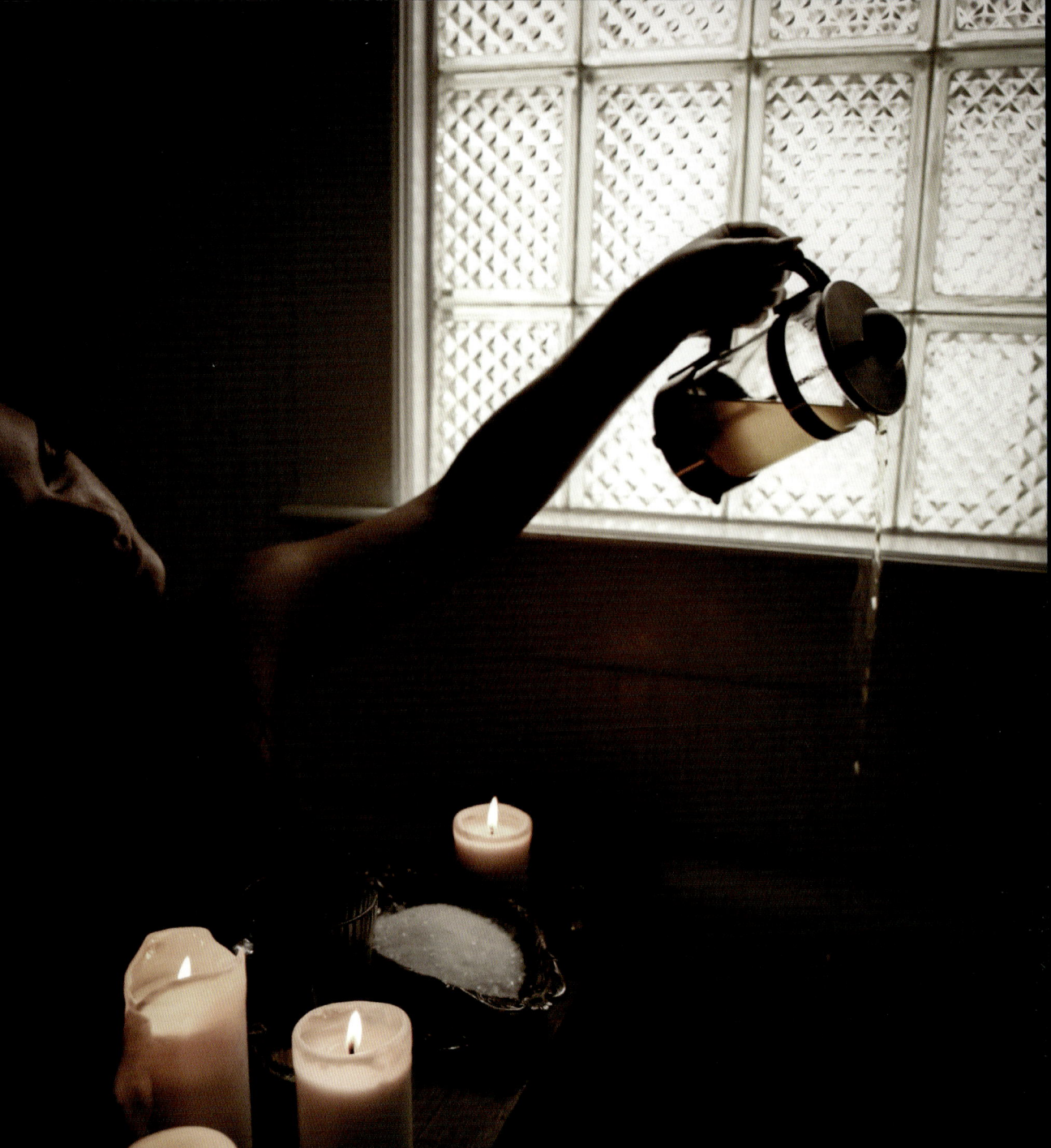

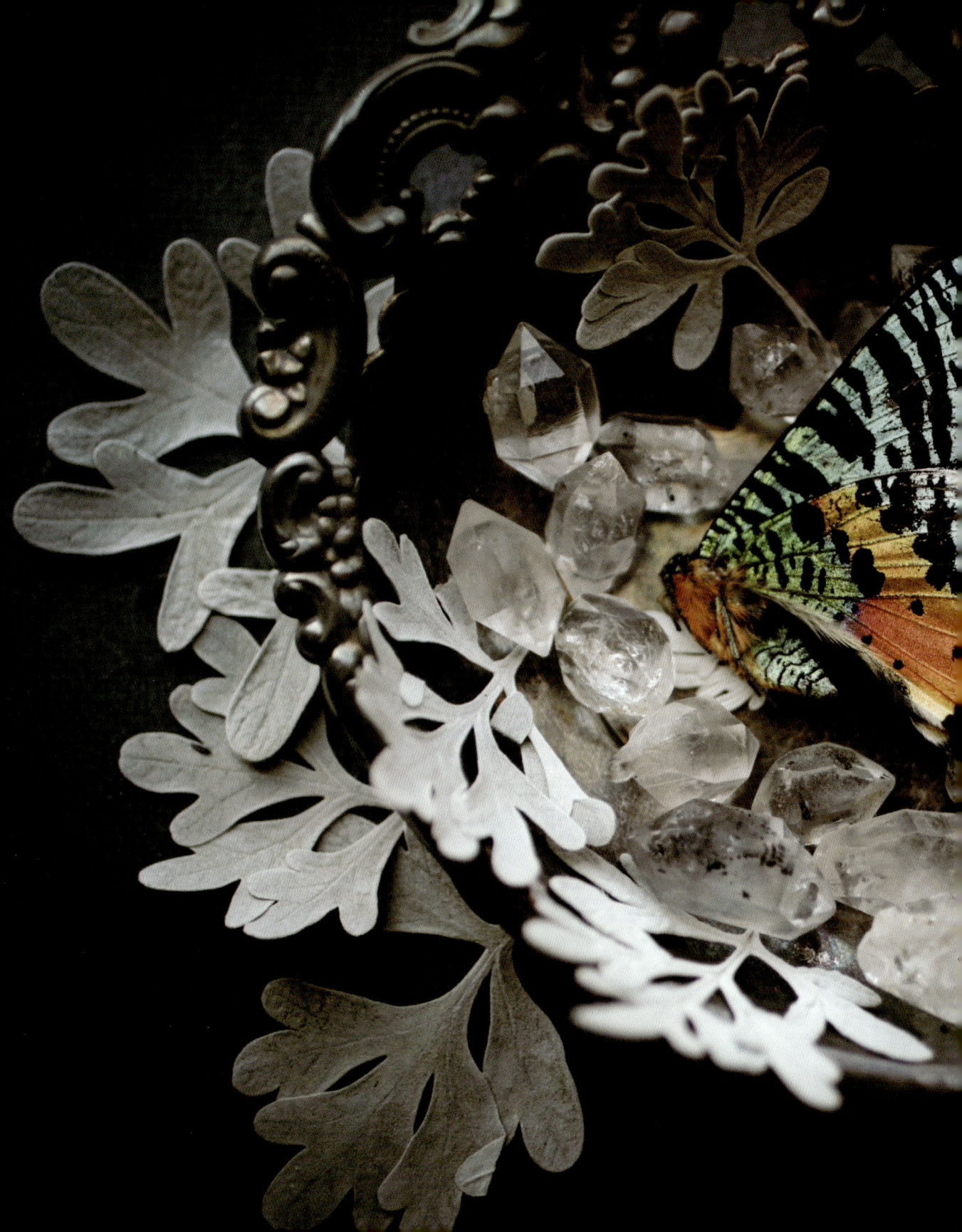

Ten

DREAM WORK

Most of what happens to us begins below the surface of consciousness, and much of what we experience is driven by what this part of our mind is programmed to see. One of the easiest ways to access our subconscious, precognitive abilities, and the creative unconscious, is through dream work.

When I was a child, I was interested in lucid dreaming. I learned to focus on something I intended to find before I fell asleep, and once my dream began, my mind would begin searching for the object within the dream. Eventually, I was able to lucidly take control of the treasure hunt.

When I was a teenager, I kept a dream journal, and I found that if I woke up out of a dream and wrote it down right away, I could remember the dream vividly throughout the day. The more I wrote down my dreams, the better I was able to recall them well after I had woken up; it was as though the journaling was retraining my brain. Soon my memories of dreams and waking life began to merge, weighing equally on my thoughts and feelings. I would sometimes discover meanings and even precognitions about my waking life within the dreams.

Later, I began to focus less on lucidity and recall and more on creating changes and relaying messages to others in my waking life. I even experimented with solving certain problems within the dreams. Instead of using a journal to record the dreams, I wrote letters to the inner layers of my consciousness before I fell asleep.

Using herbal infusions or aromatherapy mists with peppermint or rosemary before sleep helps to wake up the lucid part of our minds once we have begun dreaming.

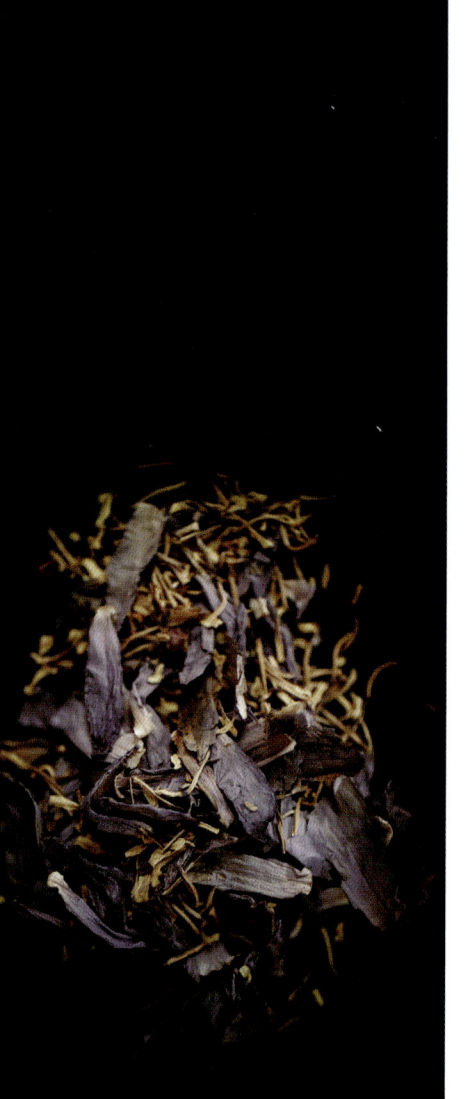

Finally, I began to study herbalism. As I explored the effects plants had on my dream work, I was able to expand upon the methods and rituals included in my nightly routine. The following dream work guide includes some of the practices that have led to significant growth in my inner world.

Dream Work Guide

For the best results with these methods, avoid regular consumption of coffee, alcohol, and any other mind-altering substances. If you are able to, it's also helpful to avoid prescription medications as well. (Note: Always consult your physician before stopping any medication.) *Do* drink green or black tea in the morning. Tea leaves contain the amino acid L-theanine, which heightens intuition and enhances dream states.

Engage in any (or all) of the following rituals before settling into sleep.

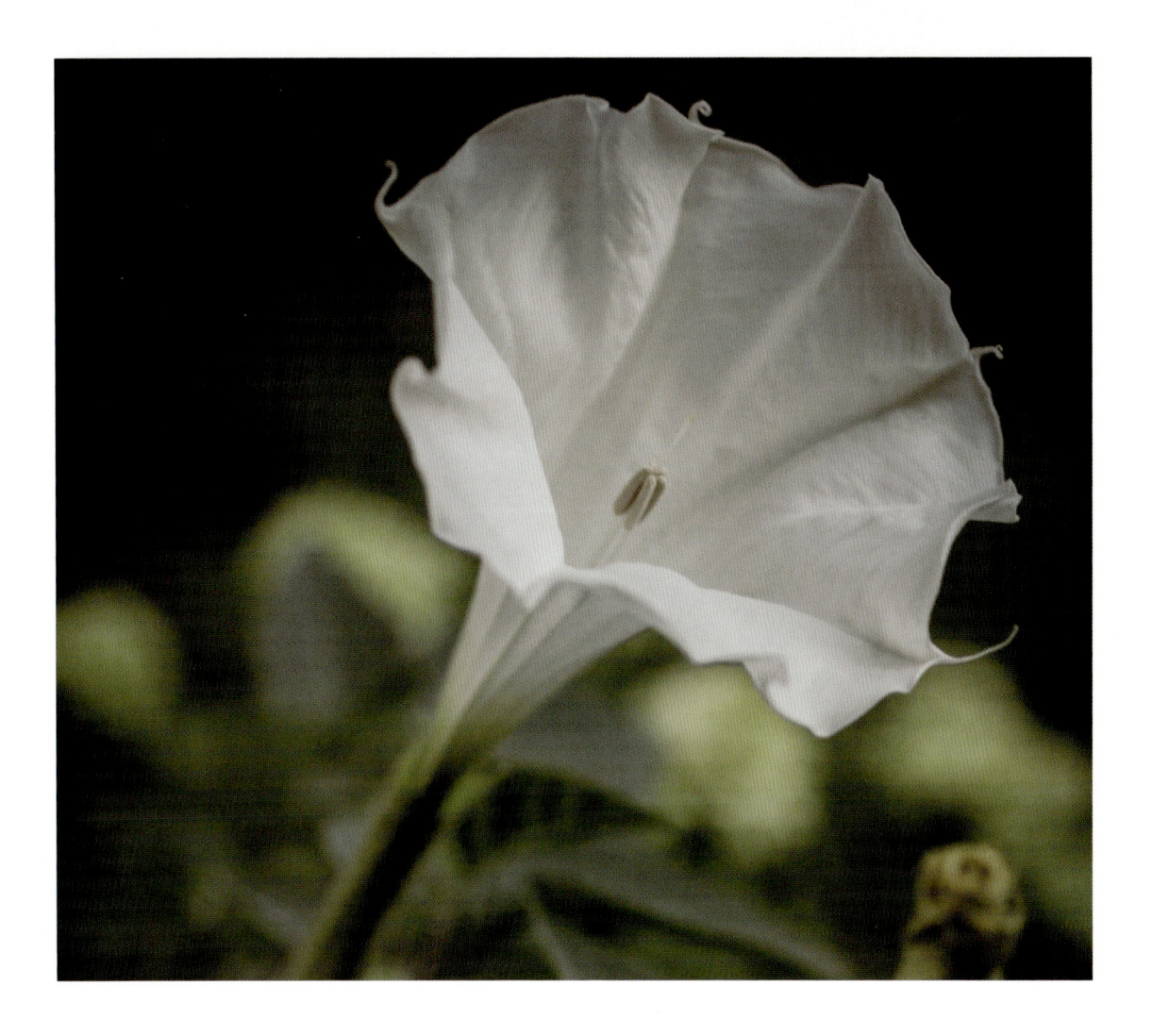

Finding Inspiration

I am often asked where I find inspiration. Inspiration comes to me when I slow down and think deeply into something. For me, it is a process of going inside instead of outside. I find the subtler details and overlooked elements are often the most fascinating. Before I fall asleep, I write down a concept I want to explore on a deeper level on paper, or I visualize it in my mind. When I wake up in the morning, I am often able to hold on to some of the visions and messages I accessed while sleeping. Having a pen and notebook nearby is useful, as well as some built-in time to document those last trailing vines from the dream realm.

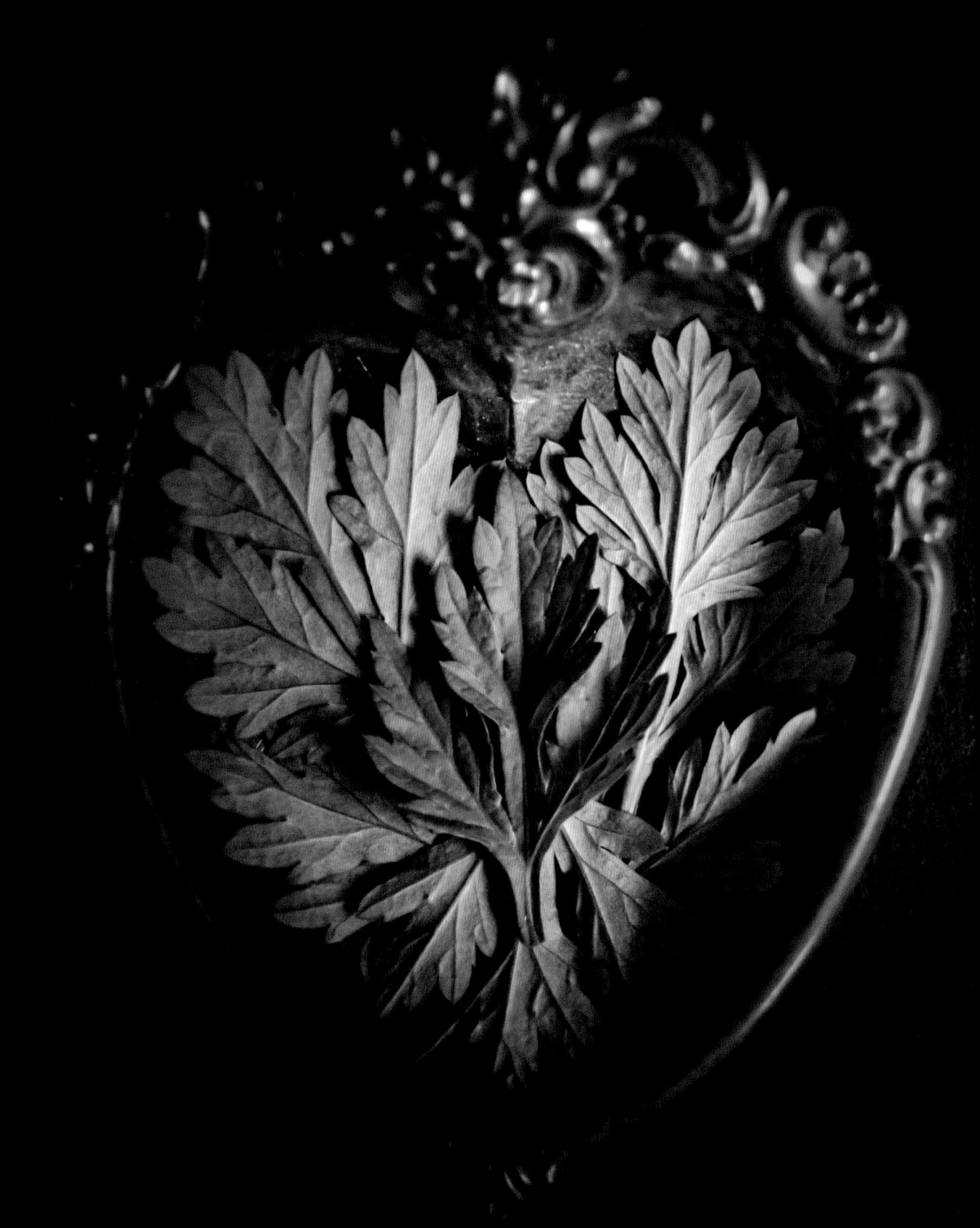

MUGWORT AND HERBAL TISANE

Thirty minutes before sleep, burn some dried mugwort over charcoal, allowing the smoke to create a soft atmosphere. Another option is to pull a small pinch of wool from a moxa stick—a therapeutic treatment from Chinese medicine made from mugwort—and place it in a dish as it burns through. (Note: Mugwort is a mild psychedelic and should be used with caution. Do not use while pregnant or before driving.)

Drink an herbal tisane containing any of the following: lemon balm, peppermint, mugwort, blue lotus, skullcap, passionflower, chamomile, tulsi, and valerian. You may want to experiment with each of these herbs on their own first, then combine them in different ways to find the right blend for you.

Lemon balm and tulsi calm the nervous system.

Blue lotus and **mugwort** enhance perception and vivify dreams.

Peppermint is relaxing to the body and stimulating to the inner mind.

Skullcap, passionflower, and **chamomile** affect the GABA (gamma-aminobutyric acid) levels in our brain, making it easier for the mind to relax. (If falling asleep isn't an issue, I recommend skipping these, as they can also suppress dreams if overused.)

Valerian root is sometimes helpful for sleep, although it can be quite strong and may induce sleep paralysis. This might be useful for astral projection work, which involves freeing your mind from your body and lucidly traveling while in a semiconscious state.

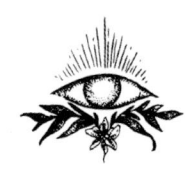

LUCID DREAM RITUAL BATH

The magnesium salt used in this bath relaxes muscles, allowing the body to rest more deeply and opening the gateway to our dreams. California poppy calms the nervous system, lavender encourages relaxation through the olfactory, mugwort enhances dreams, and peppermint keeps us lucid. Finally, activated charcoal detoxifies, removing impurities and adding a dark tint to the bathwater.

2 tablespoons dried mugwort (or 1 cup fresh)

1 tablespoon dried peppermint (or ½ cup fresh)

20 ounces filtered water (or 30 ounces if using fresh herbs)

Honey

½ teaspoon activated charcoal powder

2 milliliters (about 60 drops) California poppy tincture*

5 drops organic lavender essential oil

½ cup Dead Sea salt

1 cup Epsom salt (magnesium sulfate)

*This tincture is available in most herb shops, but you can also make your own by tincturing the seeds of this flower (see "How to Tincture," page 8).

Place the mugwort and the peppermint in a French press. Boil the filtered water and pour over the herbs; let steep for 5 to 10 minutes. Run a warm bath while this tisane infuses.

Add most of the tisane to the bathwater, saving a small cup to drink with the honey.

Mix the charcoal powder, poppy tincture, and lavender essential oil into the Dead Sea and Epsom salts. Add the salt mixture to the bathwater.

Incorporate candles, crystals, music, flowers, and incense as you wish. Soak in this bath before going to sleep, forming your dream work intentions.

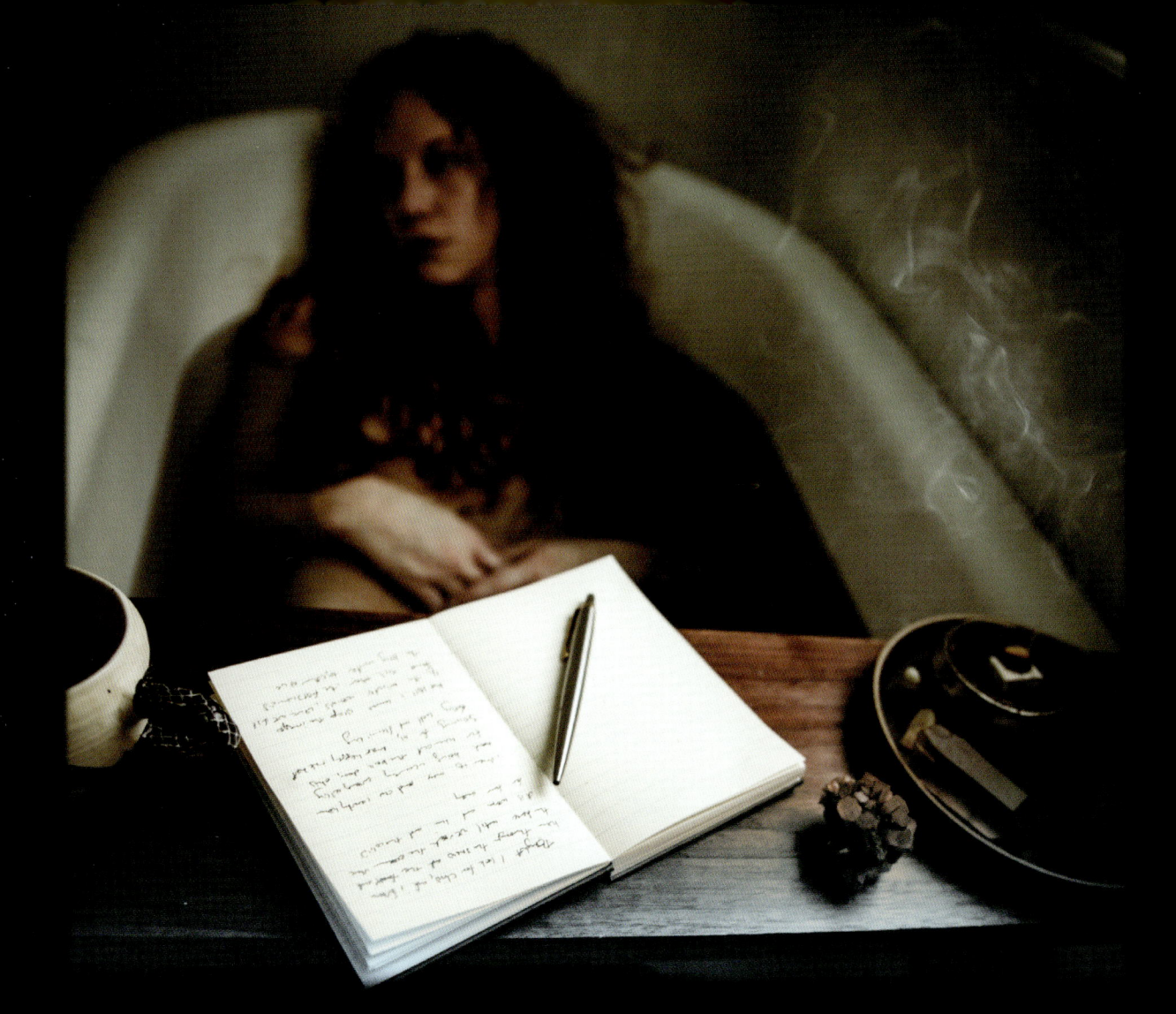

Suggested Intentions for Dream Work

Here are some examples of how to form your dream work intentions. Just before you go to bed or as you enjoy your ritual bath, write down or simply visualize the questions you want answered or the messages you want relayed in your sleep.

What do I need to know about [a situation]*?*

I want to contact [person] *and tell them* [a simple message]*.*

I want to find an answer to or make a decision about [a situation]*.*

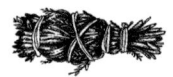

DREAM INCENSE BLEND

Makes about ½ cup of loose incense (or 27 uses)

The aromatic components of this blend are sweet and soft, relaxing the mind. The mugwort and skullcap induce lucid and prophetic dreams, and the valerian enhances astral travel capabilities. The work we do in our sleep to connect with our conscious, subconscious, and collective-conscious minds is so important, and this incense blend will guide us deeper into what we choose to seek in this state.

3 teaspoons dried mugwort

2 teaspoons ground tonka bean (or vanilla bean powder)

2 teaspoons dried lavender buds

1 teaspoon dried skullcap leaf

1 teaspoon ground valerian root

Burn all ingredients on bamboo charcoal before going to bed (see "How to Burn Loose Incense," page 71).

Breathe slowly and allow the sweet elements of this blend to infuse the atmosphere with a calming and comforting scent. You can also tincture this recipe to create a dream perfume mist for your pillow (see "How to Tincture," page 8).

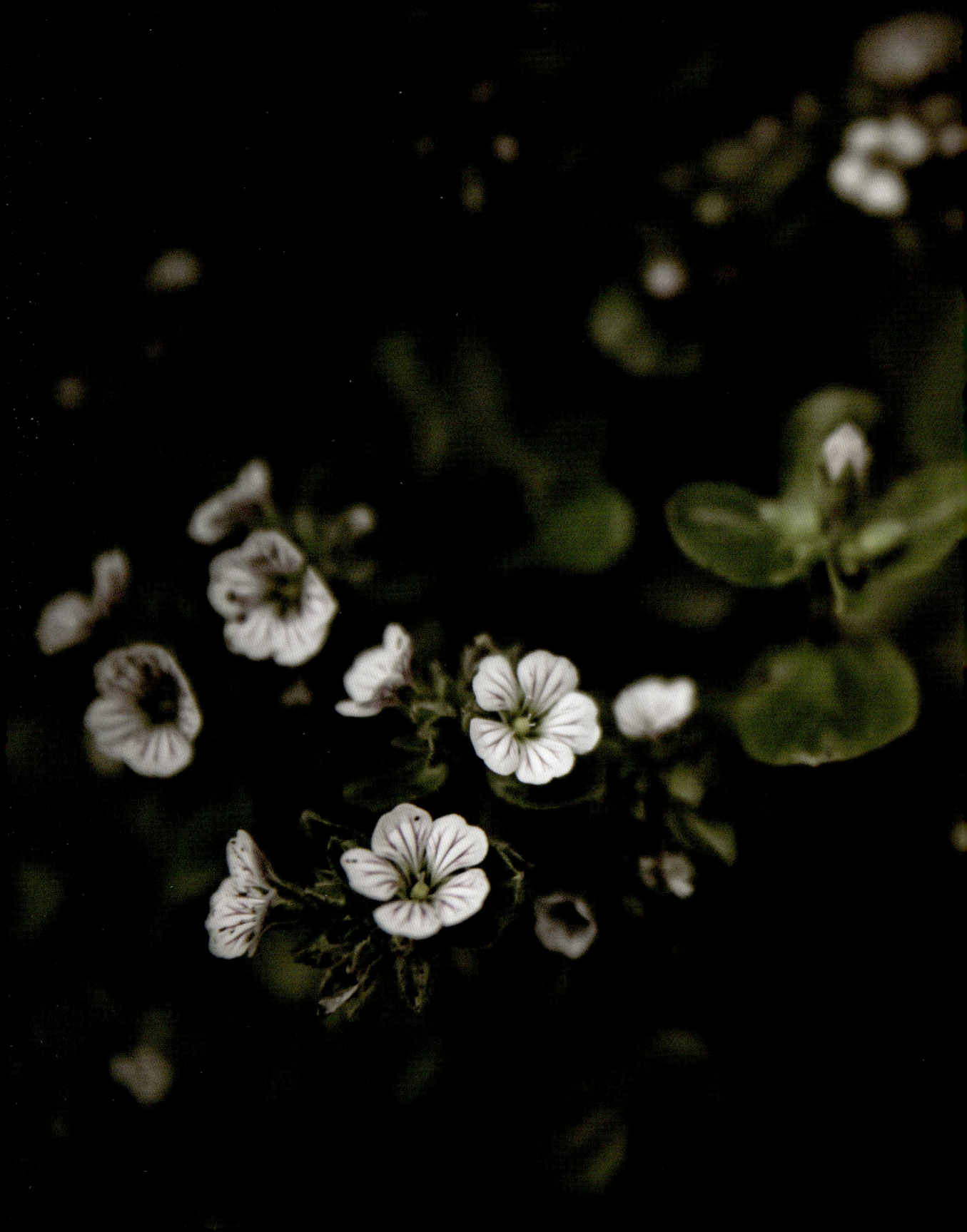

Eleven

NATURE THERAPY

Cultivating a relationship with the earth—one of appreciation and respect—is essential for remaining grounded. Despite our efforts to isolate ourselves from the forest and our feral intuition, we are still animals living in nature, and the more dependent we become on synthetic environments and technologies, the more vulnerable we are to stress, anxiety, and illness.

Grounding with Nature

Addictions are essentially habitual escapes from stress and unprocessed emotional trauma. There are a lot of ways to escape, and some of them are more socially acceptable than others. Some damage our brains and bodies, some damage our relationships to others and to ourselves, and some are detrimental to the environment. Over the years, I have learned to practice several nature-based alternatives to common, often damaging, coping strategies. While these activities are safer and healthier than their addictive counterparts, it's important to note that they are still only short-term solutions. Healing results from directly addressing the source of the pain. But finding healthy and grounding ways to comfort ourselves can make it easier to confront the underlying issues.

COMMON COPING MECHANISMS
AND NATURE-BASED ALTERNATIVES

comfort eating | aromatherapy, natural perfume

alcohol | herbal tisanes, natural perfume

television | birdwatching, being in nature

overwork, shopping | gardening, hiking, foraging

tobacco/smoking | natural incense, aromatherapy (energizing scents)

The nature-based strategies on the right engage some of the same senses, even some of the same neurotransmitters, as those on the left. The difference is in how they leave us feeling afterward: The activities on the left, while satisfying in the moment, often leave us feeling worse, while those on the right offer a sense of well-being without the negative consequences. For instance, drinking wine is both stimulating (sugar) and relaxing (alcohol), and it can offer a complex olfactory experience. Herbal tisanes can create the same effect in a more subtle way that leaves us feeling nourished instead of depleted. Likewise, smoking tobacco is stimulating and it can reduce stress because it induces a slower, deeper breathing pattern. I have found that burning a beautiful, natural incense material or inhaling an essential oil or natural perfume are the only ways I remember to slow and deepen my breath. This alone is stress reducing, and if the scents used are on the stimulating spectrum (such as mint, palo santo, or citrus), they can awaken and enliven us as well.

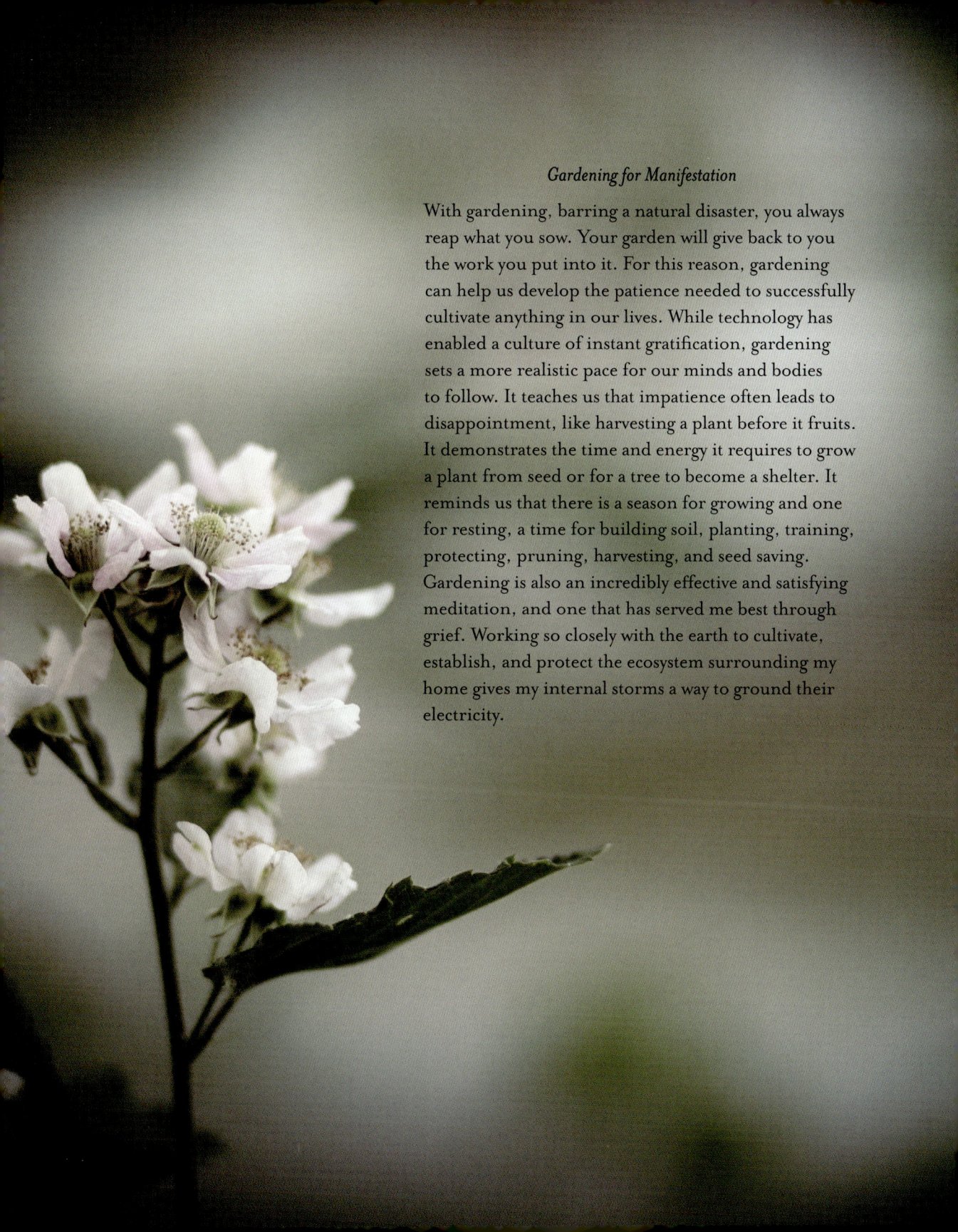

Gardening for Manifestation

With gardening, barring a natural disaster, you always reap what you sow. Your garden will give back to you the work you put into it. For this reason, gardening can help us develop the patience needed to successfully cultivate anything in our lives. While technology has enabled a culture of instant gratification, gardening sets a more realistic pace for our minds and bodies to follow. It teaches us that impatience often leads to disappointment, like harvesting a plant before it fruits. It demonstrates the time and energy it requires to grow a plant from seed or for a tree to become a shelter. It reminds us that there is a season for growing and one for resting, a time for building soil, planting, training, protecting, pruning, harvesting, and seed saving. Gardening is also an incredibly effective and satisfying meditation, and one that has served me best through grief. Working so closely with the earth to cultivate, establish, and protect the ecosystem surrounding my home gives my internal storms a way to ground their electricity.

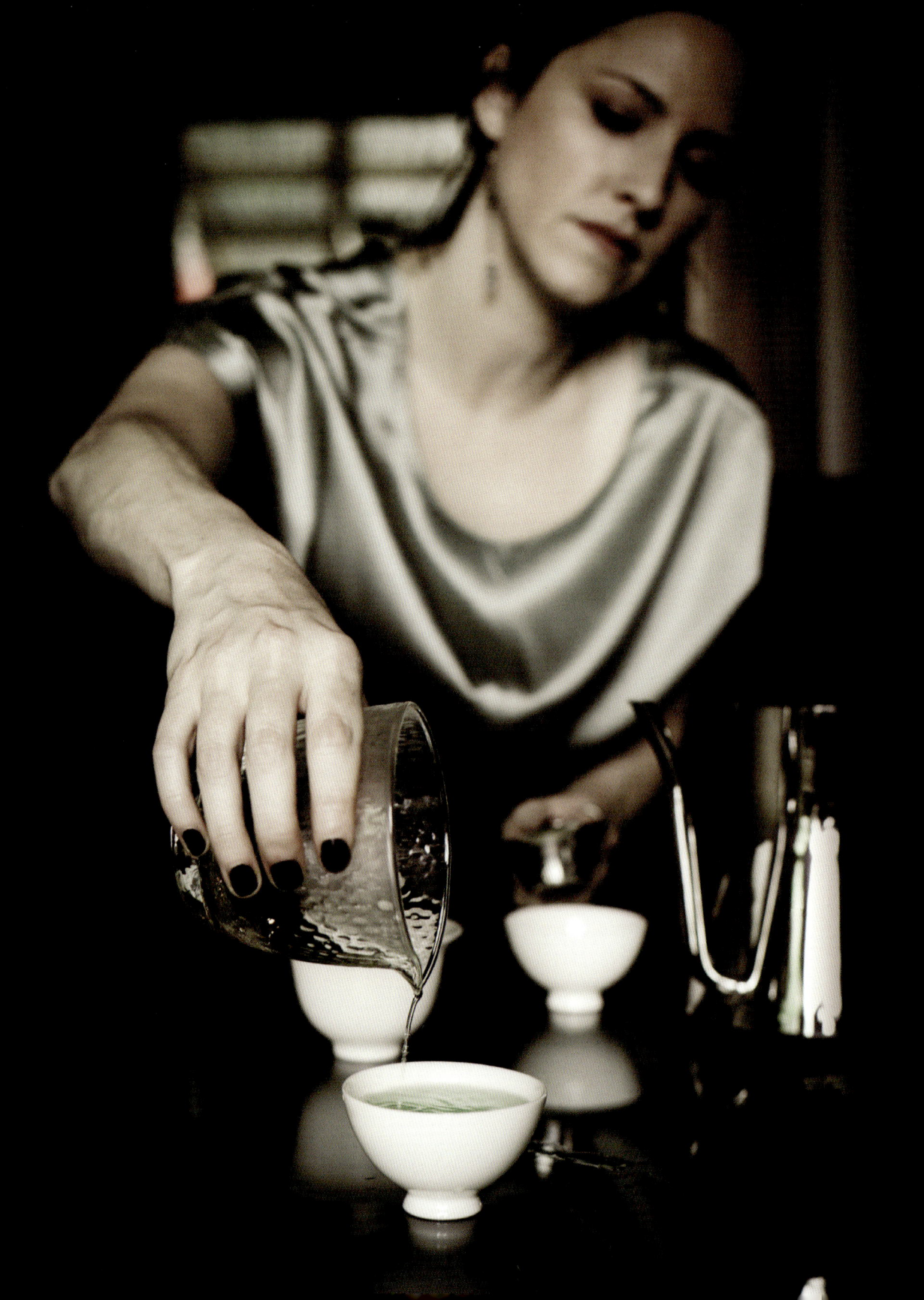

Goodbye

The recipes in this book are creative experiments and comforting rituals that I have developed over many years of working with aromatic plants. Because the work I do is so closely intertwined with my spirituality and lifestyle, I have previously kept these personal recipes and methods private, but this book has become an opportunity to be more open and to share with you some of my inner world. I hope the tools I've written about will help attune you to your senses and guide you along your journey toward developing a closer relationship with nature. I hope they inspire you to create your own meaningful connections to plants and even branch out to find other natural materials that speak to you personally. I encourage you to experiment in your own garden, kitchen, work, and even dreams, and I ask that the creative recipes I have shared with you here be reserved for personal use.

Aromatic plant essences are the spirits of botany, and they speak directly to our emotional center. The concepts of extracting them, trapping them in a bottle, mixing them together to create a new aesthetic, and wearing them are, in themselves, very strange. I'm sure the plants think so, too. As you work with plants and are comforted by their magic, always remember to reciprocate by giving back to the earth.

Suggestions for Further Reading

AROMATHERAPY AND ESSENTIAL OILS

Essential Oil Safety by Robert Tisserand and Rodney Young

Essential Oils: A Handbook for Aromatherapy Practice, 2nd Edition by Jennifer Peace Rhind

The Fragrant Mind: Aromatherapy for Personality, Mind, Mood, and Emotion
by Valerie Ann Worwood

HYDROSOLS

Harvest to Hydrosol: Distill Your Own Exquisite Hydrosols at Home by Ann Harmon

BOTANICAL PERFUME

Essence & Alchemy: A Natural History of Perfume by Mandy Aftel

Perfume and Flavor Materials of Natural Origin by Steffen Arctander

HERBALISM

Herbal Recipes for Vibrant Health by Rosemary Gladstar

Herbs & Things by Jeanne Rose

Planetary Herbology: An Integration of Western Herbs into the Traditional Chinese and Ayurvedis Systems by Michael Tierra, C.A., N.D.

MOON PHASES

Llewellyn's *Moon Sign Book*

Moon Magic by Lori Reid

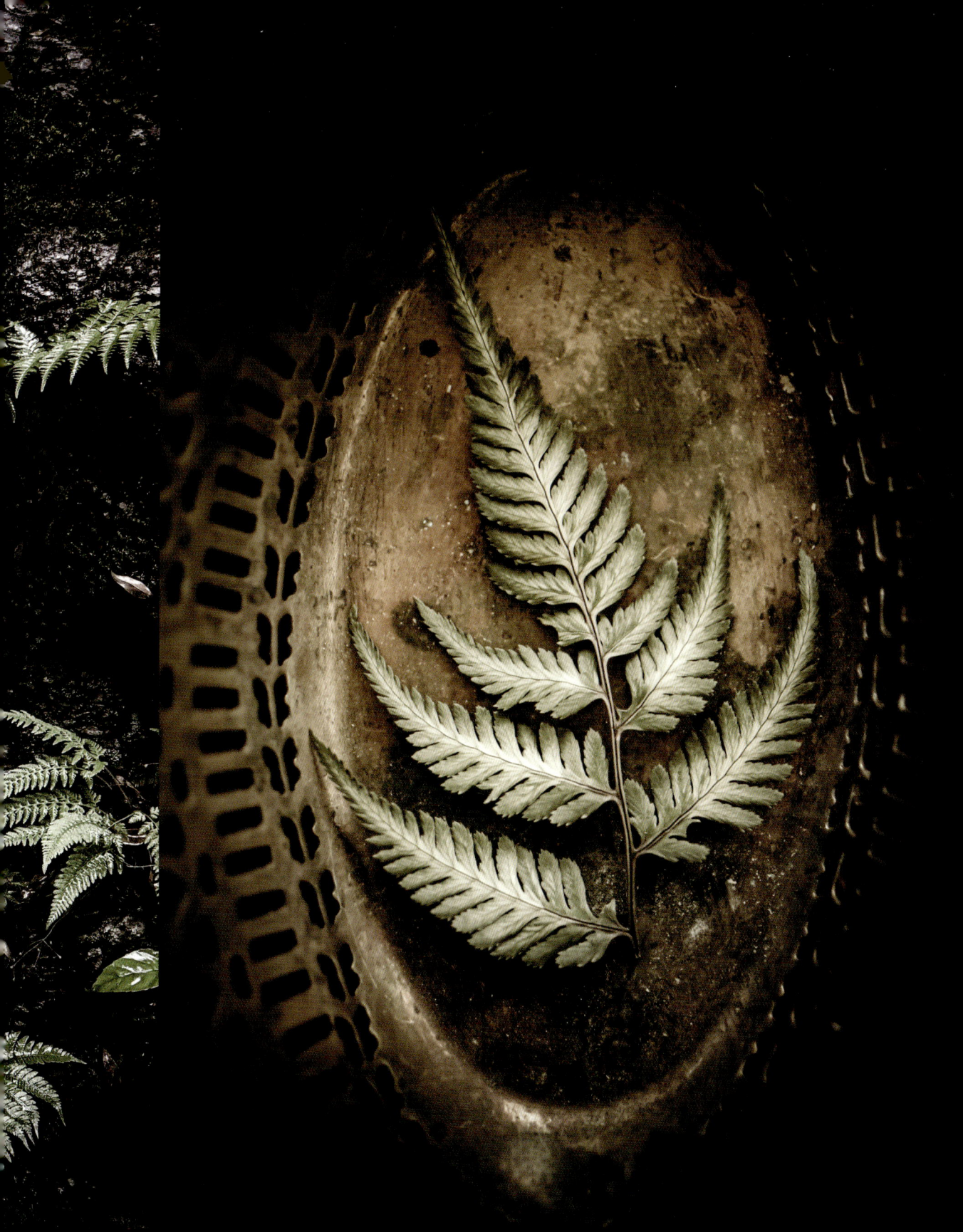

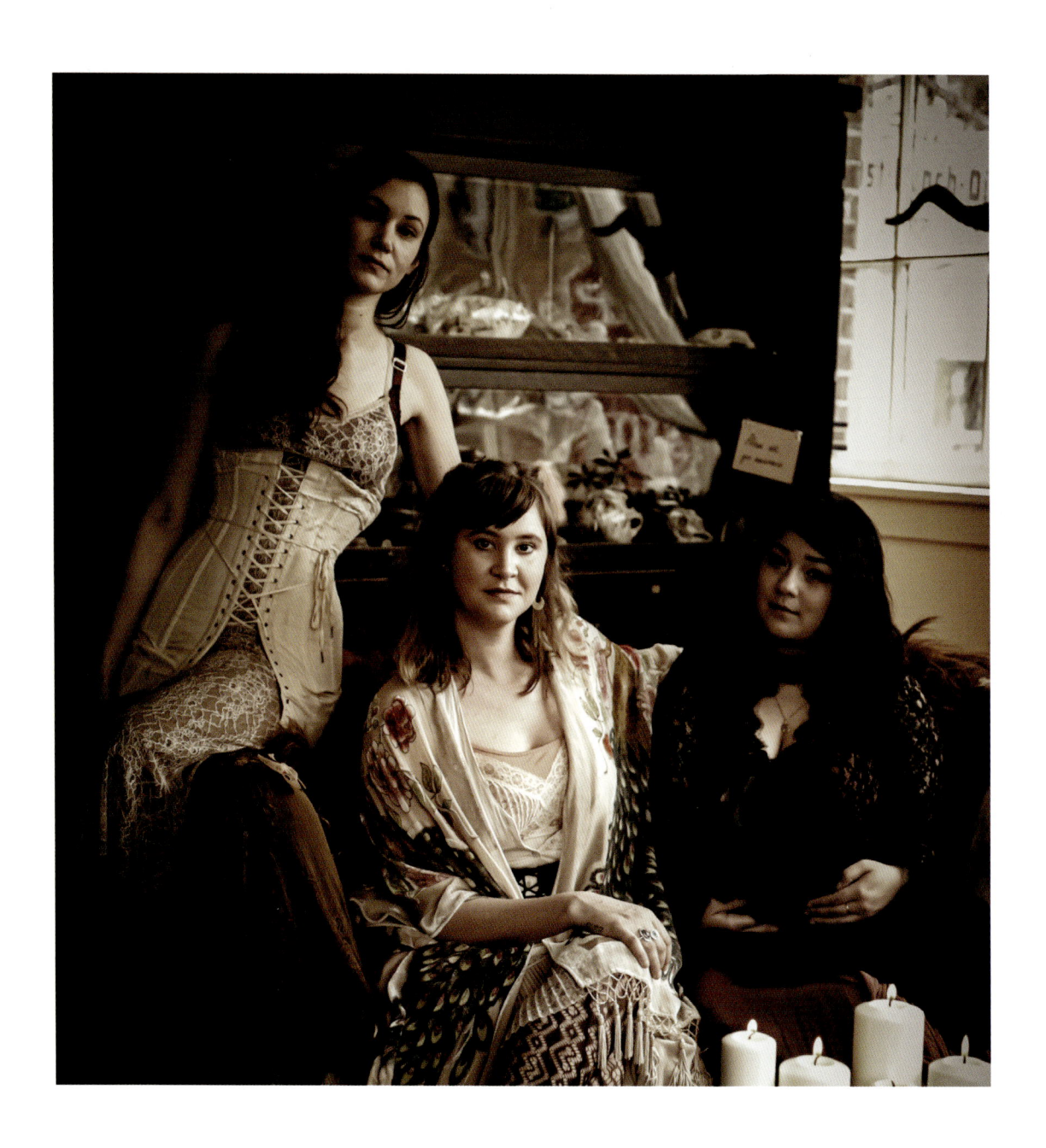

Acknowledgments

Thank you so much to my friends and family who have been involved with this work. To Luke and Jennifer Wetzel for igniting the idea for this book and encouraging it, and to the crew—Tara Milleville, Ash Miyagawa, and Ruby Hanson—for contributing your love and talent to For Strange Women.

About the Author

Jill McKeever is the creator of the independent perfume house For Strange Women. She works exclusively with natural materials, developing a synesthetic approach to scent from the realm of sound. In 2009, she combined her perfume technique with her photography, design, and writing to capture a devoted online following. Jill continues to explore the aesthetic, therapeutic, and esoteric qualities of the plants that compose the perfumes she constructs in her studio.

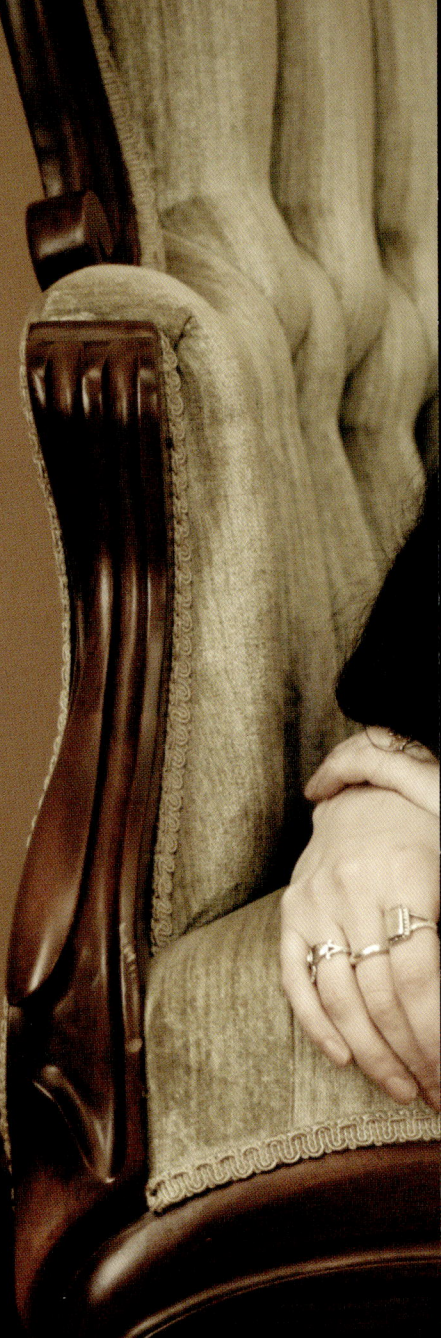

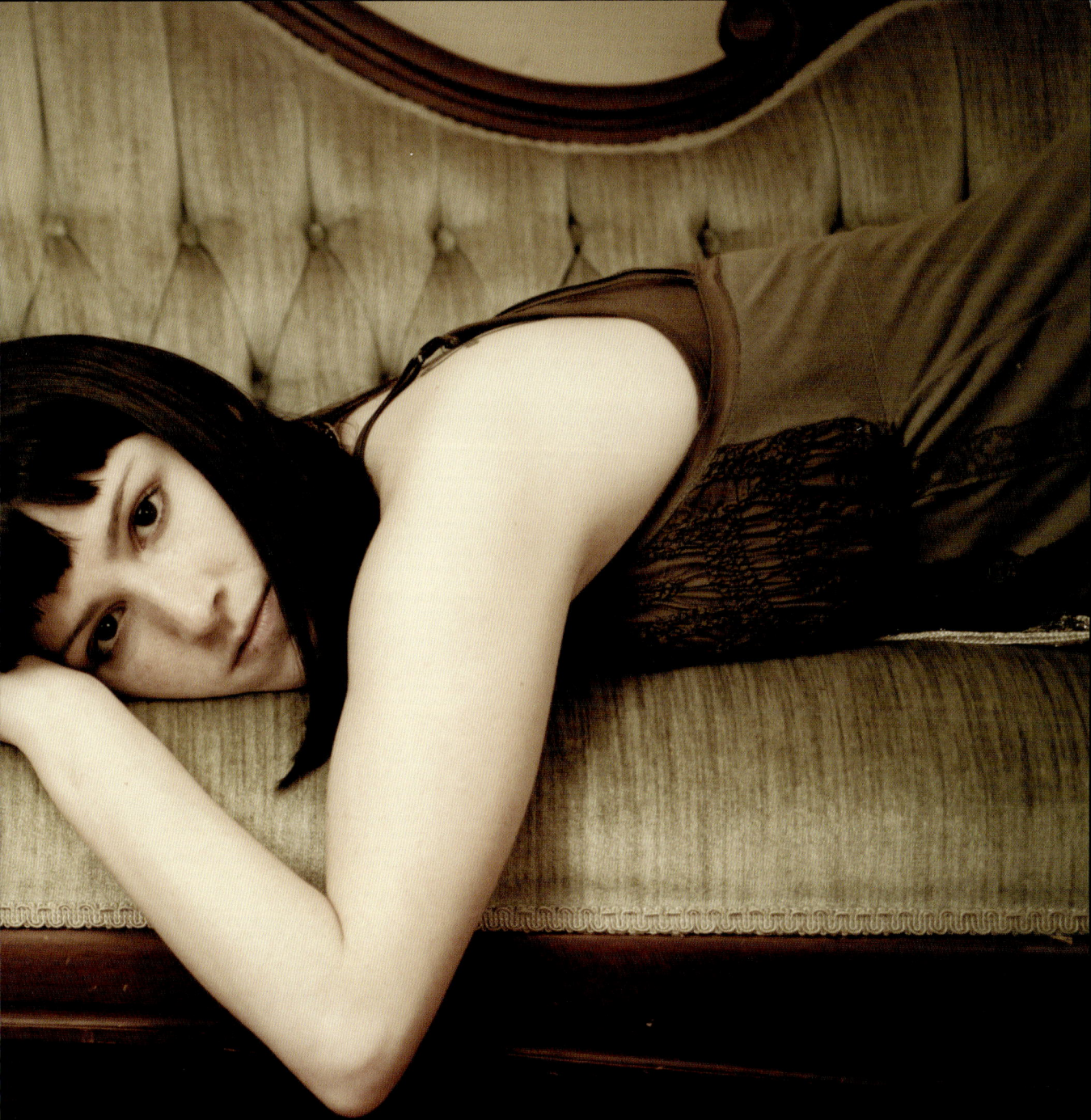

Index

— A —

agarwood, 54, 103, 115
amber, 115, 116
angelica, 59, 60
Anti-Anxiety Aromatherapy Inhaler, 102
antioxidant, 34
anxiety, 51, 55, 101, 103, 131
    Anti-Anxiety Aromatherapy Inhaler, 102
    Full Moon Guided Trance, 96
Aquarius astrological sign, 116
Aries astrological sign, 113
aromatherapy, ix, 11, 101, 120
    Anti-Anxiety Aromatherapy Inhaler, 102
    blends for, 106–7
    botanical perfume and, 25
    geographical scentscapes for, 107–11
    Healing Roots Aromatherapy Inhaler, 60
    home integration of, 104
    hydrosols and, 41
    as nature-based alternative, 132
    roots and, 59
    scent horoscopes, 112–16
aromatics, ix. *See also* essential oils
    component characteristics, 13
    extracted, 1, 2, 4
    relationship with, 14–15
    and botanical perfume, 24–25
    sound and, 27–31
    as spirits of botany, 135
Artemisia tridentata. See big sagebrush
astrology
    Aquarius, 116
    Aries, 113
    Cancer, 114
    Capricorn, 116
    Gemini, 113
    Leo, 114
    Libra, 115
    Pisces, 116
    Sagittarius, 115
    scent horoscopes, 112–16
    Scorpio, 115
    Taurus, 113
    Virgo, 115
attack, of scents, 29
autumn, 79
    Autumn Equinox Loose Incense, 80
    Autumn-inspired diffusion blend, 81

— B —

balms and salves
    London Fog Lip Balm, 37–39
    Vetiver Healing Salve, 62–63
balsam, 113, 116
baths, 2
    Lucid Dream Ritual Bath, 124–25
    Winter Solstice Ritual Bath, 84–85
bergamot, 6, 33, 37, 55, 56, 81, 107
beverages. *See* teas and beverages
big sagebrush (*Artemisia tridentata*), 72, 73, 75, 76
blackberry leaves, 91
blue lotus, 123
borage, 91
botanical perfume, 1, 4–7, 23
    aromatherapy and, 25
    attack of, 29
    Calming Perfume Mist, 49–50
    chorus effects of, 30
    map for, 31
    musical terms for, 27–30
    not cosmetic, 21–22
    notes of, 25, 27
    Palo Santo Energy-Unblocking Perfume, 56–58
    production of, 25
    release in, 30
    reverberation in, 28
    scent equalization in, 29
    scent memories and, 25
    selection of, 24–25
    spirit realm and, 22
    Spring Equinox Perfume, 88–89
    synthetic perfume compared with, 21
    waveforms of, 29
Bursera graveolens. See palo santo

— C —

California poppy, 124–25
Calming Perfume Mist, 49–50
Cancer astrological sign, 114
Capricorn astrological sign, 116
cardamom
    Cardamom and Spruce Tea, 34–35
    how to use, 34
cedar, 18, 52, 84. *See also* Eastern red cedar
chamomile, 91, 107, 123
charcoals, 71, 75, 80, 108, 111, 124–25, 127
China, 111
chorus effects, 30
citrus, 17, 18, 33, 55, 107, 113, 114, 132
clary sage, 49–50, 95, 96–97, 104. *See also* sage
cleaning supplies, 99
cocoa, 114
coconut milk, 84–85
Colorado, 107
confirmation ceremony, 2

coping mechanisms, 131–32
coumarin, 49
creative unconscious, 119, 129
creativity, 107, 129
cypress, 102

— D —

dance, 1, 4, 23
deserts, 72, 111
diffusers. *See* mists and diffusers
dream work
    Dream Incense Blend, 127
    guide for, 120
    and inspiration, 121
    intentions for, 126
    Lucid Dream Ritual Bath, 124–25
    Mugwort and Herbal Tisane, 123
    role of, 119

— E —

Earl Grey tea, 37
Earthship Bioculture, 72
Eastern red cedar (*Juniperus virginiana*)
    essential oil, 52, 76–77
    incense, 74
Epsom salt. *See* magnesium salt
essential oils, 106. *See also specific essential oils*
    batch number of, 17
    botanical name for, 17
    cautions for usage, 11–12
    cedar, 52
    considerations for blending, 13
    fragrance oil compared with, 17
    Full Moon Botanical Trance Oil, 95–97
    health claims and, 16
    home integration of, 104
    ingredients, 18
    organic, 16
    packaging and storage of, 17
    purchase guidelines for, 16–18
    quantity of, 18
    relationship with, 13–15
    for soaps, 104
    source of, 18
    spirit realm and, 2, 4
    sustainability of, 18
eucalyptus, 102, 104, 107, 114
evergreen needles, 34, 114

— F —

fir, 84–85, 102, 104
first quarter moon/waxing gibbous, 94
flowers, 8, 15, 25, 40, 79, 125. *See also specific flowers*
For Strange Women perfume house, 13, 27, 93, 139, 140
forests, 111
frankincense, 6–7, 45, 56–57, 62–63, 64, 80, 88–89, 107, 111, 115
full moon, 94
    Full Moon Botanical Trance Oil, 95
    Full Moon Guided Trance, 96–97

— G —

gamma-aminobutyric acid (GABA), 123
gardenia, 114
gardening, 15, 25, 132, 133
gas chromatography/mass spectrometry (GCMS), 17
Gemini astrological sign, 113
geographical scentscapes
    for aromatherapy, 107–11
    deserts, 111
    mountains, 107–9
    oceans, 111
    temperate deciduous forests, 111
ginger, 59, 107, 114
grapefruit, 6–7, 33, 107
grasses, 48. *See also* sweetgrass
guided trance, 96–97

— H —

Healing Roots Aromatherapy Inhaler, 60
Herbal Tisane, 123, 132
herbalism, 8, 11, 120
hops, 107
HVAC diffusion method, 102, 104
hydrosols, 40, 41, 42, 44, 56, 88, 104
hypothalamus, 11

— I —

incense, 2, 115
    Autumn Equinox Loose Incense, 80
    big sagebrush, 73, 75
    Dream Incense Blend, 127
    Eastern red cedar, 74
    homemade, 69
    how to burn, 71
    Incense Blend for Spirit Cleansing, Protection, and Strength, 75, 111
    Mountain Incense, 108–9
    mugwort, 123
    palo santo, 53, 55, 73, 75
    for psychic protection, 73
    resins for, 64, 65
    respect for, 70
    sweetgrass, 74, 75
    synthetic, 69
    woods for, 103
    yerba santa, 74, 75
India, 34, 60
infusions, 2, 8, 120
    New Moon Cleaning Infusion, 99
    whole-herb-infused waters, 12
inhalers, 59, 106
    Anti-Anxiety Aromatherapy Inhaler, 102
    Healing Roots Aromatherapy Inhaler, 60
inspiration, 1, 13, 22, 33, 98, 121, 129, 135

J

Japan, 70, 103
jasmine, 6–7, 14, 104, 107, 111, 114, 115
jojoba oil, 18, 62, 95
Juniperus virginiana. See Eastern red cedar

K

Kombu Tincture, 6–7

L

last quarter moon, 98
lavender, 6–7, 18, 88–89, 95–97, 99, 104, 107, 108, 111, 113, 116, 124–25, 127
    Lavender and Sage Tea, 45–47
    Lavender Lemonade, 43
    Lavender Tincture, 43, 49–50
leather, 115
lemon balm, 91, 123
lemongrass, 48
Leo astrological sign, 114
Libra astrological sign, 115
limbic system, 23, 69
lime, 111
Lucid Dream Ritual Bath, 124–25
London Fog Lip Balm, 37–39
L-theanine, 120

M

magnesium salt, 84–85, 124–25
may chang, 107
meditation, 4, 23, 45, 60, 93, 101, 102, 103, 107, 115, 133
memory, 107
Midsummer Iced Mint Tisane, 91
mint, 90, 91, 132
mists and diffusers, 106, 108, 120
    Autumn-inspired diffusion blend, 81
    Calming Perfume Mist, 49–50
    HVAC diffusion method, 102, 104
    for pets, 104
    Psychic Cleansing Room–Linen–Body Mist, 76–77
moon
    first quarter/waxing gibbous, 94
    full moon, 94
    Full Moon Botanical Trance Oil, 95
    Full Moon Guided Trance, 96–97
    last quarter, 98
    new moon, 73, 93
    New Moon Cleaning Infusion, 99
    synchronized energy and, 93
mountains
    as geographical scentscape, 25, 107, 116
    Mountain Incense, 108–9
moxa stick, 123
mugwort, 123, 124–25, 127
music, 1, 4, 23, 85, 106, 125, 128
    terms for botanical perfume, 27–30
myrrh, 64, 111, 115

N

nature, grounding with, 131
    alternative coping mechanisms, 132
    gardening for, 133
neroli, 44, 95, 107
New Mexico, 72
new moon, 73, 93
    New Moon Cleaning Infusion, 99
notes
    of botanical perfume, 25, 27
    clean compared with musky, 113
    of resins, 64
    top notes, 5

O

oakmoss, 14, 111, 116
oceans, 93, 111
oleo-gum-resins, 65
olfactory system, 11, 21, 23, 29, 40, 124, 132
orange blossom water, 41, 56–57, 104
    Saffron and Orange Blossom Lemonade, 44
orris, 80, 107, 108, 115
oud, 54. *See* agarwood

P

palmarosa, 48
palo santo (*Bursera graveolens*), 53–55, 76–77, 107, 115, 132
    incense, 73, 75
    Palo Santo Energy-Unblocking Perfume, 56–57
    Palo Santo Tincture, 56–57
passionflower, 123
patchouli, 18, 29, 107, 115
peppermint, 18, 84–85, 91, 104, 107, 120, 123, 124–25
perfume. *See* botanical perfume
piñon, 111
Pisces astrological sign, 116
Propolis Tincture, 88–89
Psychic Cleansing Room–Linen–Body Mist, 76–77
psychic protection, 73
pu-erh tea, 111

R

Rasputina, 107
relaxation, 13, 45, 60, 84, 98, 107, 116, 123, 124, 127, 129, 132
release, 30
resins, 15, 25, 28, 30, 34, 69, 76, 113. *See also specific resins*
    incense, 64, 65
    notes of, 64
    oleo-gum, 65
    Mountain Incense, 108
    tips for, 65
reverberation, 28
rhizomes, 59
roots, 8, 15, 18. *See also specific roots*
    aromatherapy and, 59, 115

Healing Roots Aromatherapy
  Inhaler, 60
 sustainability of, 59
rose, 29, 40, 88–89, 107, 115, 116
 rose water, 40–41, 104
 Rose Water Lemonade, 42
rosemary, 6–7, 99, 104, 107, 111, 120

——— S ———

Saffron and Orange Blossom
  Lemonade, 44
sage, 45–47, 99, 107. *See also* clary sage
Sagittarius astrological sign, 115
salves. *See* balms and salves
sandalwood, 54, 102, 103, 104, 107,
  114, 115
scent equalization, 29
scent memories, 13–14, 25
scentscapes, 30
Scorpio astrological sign, 115
seashells, 111
seduction, 107
seeds, 33, 34. *See also* cardamom; *specific seeds*
skullcap, 123, 127
sleep, 107, 123, 127
smoke, 115
smudge wands, 73
soaps, 2, 21, 59, 104
spirit realm, 2, 4
spring, 86
 Spring Equinox Perfume, 88–89
strawberry leaves, 91
summer, 90, 91
sustainability, 11, 18, 40, 54, 59, 72, 93
sweet basil, 107
sweetgrass, 48
 incense, 74, 75, 76–77, 108
 Sweetgrass Tincture, 49–50
sycamore, 111
synesthesia, 27–31, 139

——— T ———

Taurus astrological sign, 113
teas and beverages, 120
 Cardamom and Spruce Tea, 34–35
 Earl Grey, 37
 Herbal Tisane, 123, 132
 Lavender and Sage Tea, 45–47
 Lavender Lemonade, 43
 Midsummer Iced Mint Tisane, 91
 pu-erh tea, 111
 Rose Water Lemonade, 42
 Saffron and Orange Blossom
  Lemonade, 44
theta brain waves, 129
third eye, 55, 56
tinctures, 108
 Kombu Tincture, 6–7
 Lavender Tincture, 43, 49–50
 Palo Santo Tincture, 56–57
 for physical health, 12
 Propolis Tincture, 88–89
 steps for making, 8, 9
 Sweetgrass Tincture, 49–50
 Tincture for Strange Women, 5,
  6–7, 111
tisane, 90, 104, 123, 124–25, 132
 Midsummer Iced Mint Tisane, 91
tobacco, 114, 132
travel, 15, 25, 107
tulsi, 91, 107, 123

——— V ———

valerian, 59, 107, 123, 127
vanilla, 36, 37–39, 49, 74, 80, 107,
  116, 127
vetiver, 60–61, 88–89
 Vetiver Healing Salve, 62–63
vinegars, 12, 99
Virgo astrological sign, 115

——— W ———

waveforms, 29
white copal, 64, 108

whole-herb-infused waters, 12
winter, 83
 Winter Solstice Ritual Bath, 84–85
woods, 34–35, 51, 52, 115. *See also*
  cedar; palo santo; *specific woods*
 incense, 103
 sustainability of, 54

——— Y ———

yerba santa, 74, 75–76
ylang-ylang, 6–7, 49–50, 107

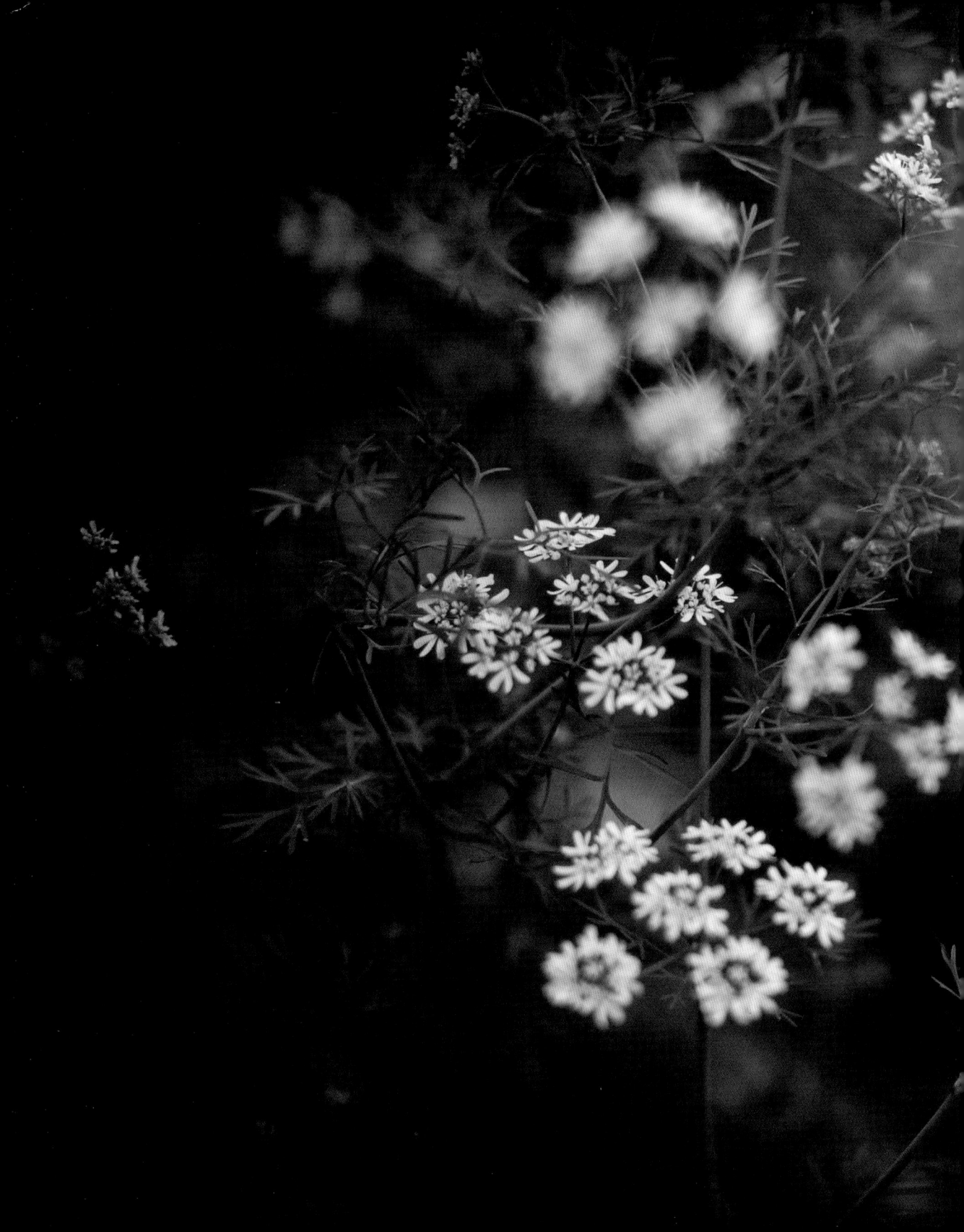

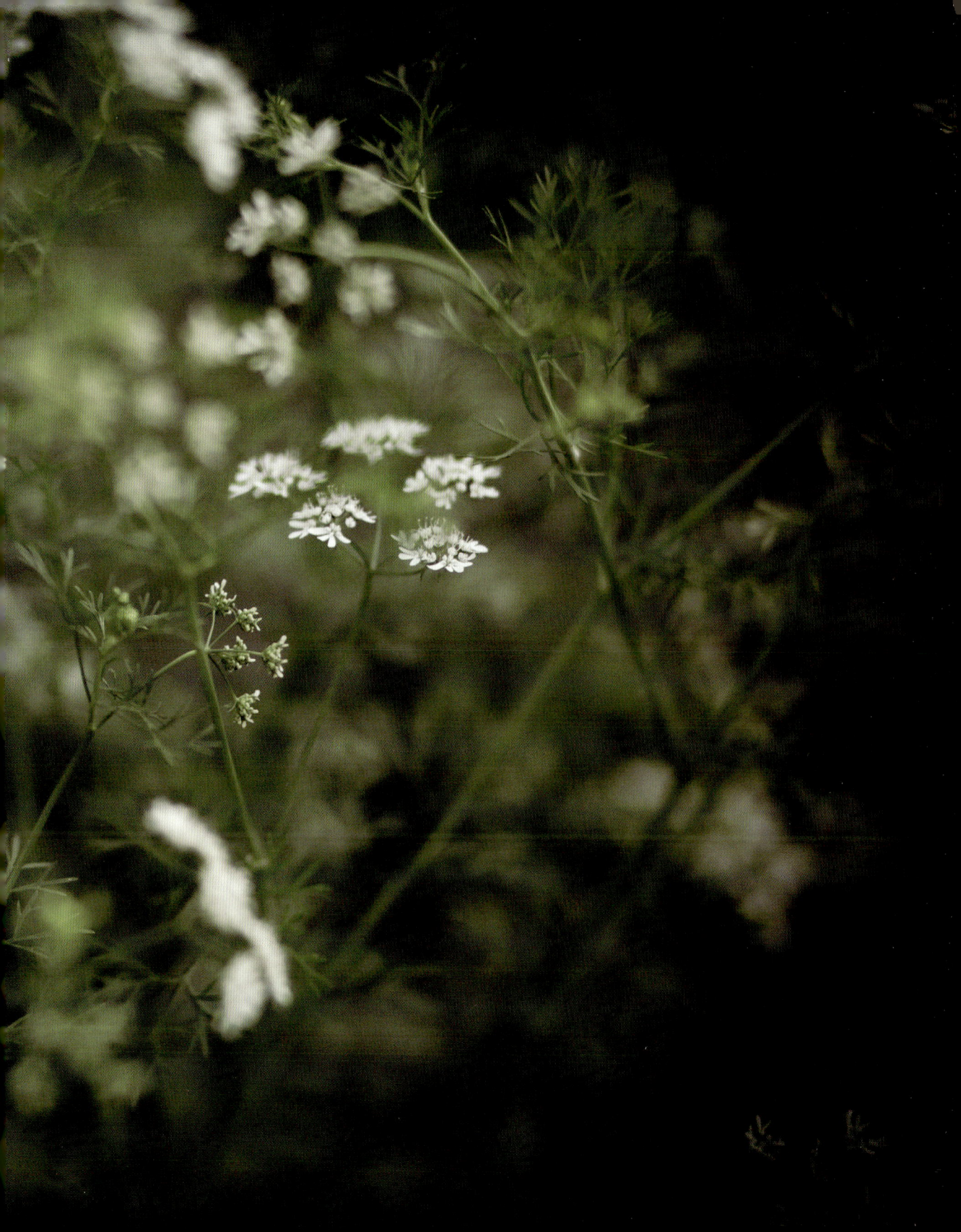

The Spirit of Botany

copyright © 2020 by Jill McKeever. All rights reserved. Printed in China.
No part of this book may be used or reproduced in any manner whatsoever without
written permission except in the case of reprints in the context of reviews.

Andrews McMeel Publishing
a division of Andrews McMeel Universal
1130 Walnut Street, Kansas City, Missouri 64106

www.andrewsmcmeel.com

20 21 22 23 24 SDB 10 9 8 7 6 5 4 3 2 1

ISBN: 978-1-5248-5459-1

Library of Congress Control Number: 2020931796

Illustrations by Ash Miyagawa
Photography by Jill McKeever and Jennifer Wetzel
Author photos (pages xii, 140) by Jessica Brothers

Editor: Melissa Rhodes Zahorsky
Art Director/Designer: Holly Swayne
Production Editor: Elizabeth A. Garcia
Production Manager: Carol Coe

ATTENTION: SCHOOLS AND BUSINESSES

Andrews McMeel books are available at quantity discounts with bulk purchase for
educational, business, or sales promotional use. For information, please e-mail the
Andrews McMeel Publishing Special Sales Department: specialsales@amuniversal.com.